Understanding the NHS

Dedication

This book is dedicated to my mother, Dr Gillian Matthews, and my late father, Dr Maurice Stein. They worked hard for their whole lives, were 100% dedicated to the NHS, and made a difference. You too, like them, can make a difference. My mother never allowed any of us to say "I can't". That is my motto too, and is my advice to you.

Finally, I would like to thank my wife Emma, and children Poppy and Isaac for putting up with me; and bringing me cups of tea and coffee, as yet again, I disappear into my office to write (another!) book.

"When the hurlyburly's done,
When the battle's lost and won."

Macbeth
Act One, Scene One

Understanding the NHS
How to Get the Most from Our National Health Service

Andy Stein

(Reviewed by Yakup Kilic and James Korolewicz)

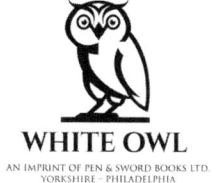

WHITE OWL
AN IMPRINT OF PEN & SWORD BOOKS LTD.
YORKSHIRE - PHILADELPHIA

First published in Great Britain in 2022 by
White Owl
An imprint of
Pen & Sword Books Ltd
Yorkshire - Philadelphia

Copyright © Andy Stein, 2022

ISBN 978 1 39900 796 2

The right of Andy Stein to be identified as author of this work has been asserted by him in accordance with the Copyright, Designs and Patents Act 1988.

A CIP catalogue record for this book is available from the British Library.

All rights reserved. No part of this book may be reproduced or transmitted in any form or by any means, electronic or mechanical including photocopying, recording or by any information storage and retrieval system, without permission from the Publisher in writing.

Typeset in Times New Roman 10/13 by SJmagic DESIGN SERVICES, India.

Printed and bound in the Uk by CPI Group (UK) Ltd., Croydon. CR0 4YY.

Pen & Sword Books Ltd incorporates the imprints of Pen & Sword Books Archaeology, Atlas, Aviation, Battleground, Discovery, Family History, History, Maritime, Military, Naval, Politics, Railways, Select, Transport, True Crime, Fiction, Frontline Books, Leo Cooper, Praetorian Press, Seaforth Publishing, Wharncliffe and White Owl.

For a complete list of Pen & Sword titles please contact

PEN & SWORD BOOKS LIMITED
47 Church Street, Barnsley, South Yorkshire, S70 2AS, England
E-mail: enquiries@pen-and-sword.co.uk
Website: www.pen-and-sword.co.uk

or

PEN AND SWORD BOOKS
1950 Lawrence Rd, Havertown, PA 19083, USA
E-mail: Uspen-and-sword@casematepublishers.com
Website: www.penandswordbooks.com

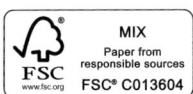

Contents

Acknowledgements vi

Foreword vii

Introduction ix

Chapter 1   History of NHS: Beginning and Consolidation 1

Chapter 2   History of NHS: Modernisation 14

Chapter 3   Services, Buildings and Funding 27

Chapter 4   Staff and Training 48

Chapter 5   Organisations 71

Chapter 6   Specialists and Specialised Commissioning 86

Chapter 7   Mental Health 98

Chapter 8   Public Health 111

Chapter 9   Research 129

Chapter 10   The Digital NHS 146

Chapter 11   Sorting out the NHS 162

Chapter 12   The Future of the NHS 179

Chapter 13   Glossary and Acronym-Buster 193

Chapter 14   History of NHS Summary 217

Index 222

Acknowledgements

Many colleagues assisted in the writing of this book. It was a team effort. I am very grateful to the following people, who worked on the chapters indicated:

- Rebekah Harris, Lucy Brecker and Jon Franklin (History of NHS);
- Titilope Omitogun, Saidya Najeeb; Andy Beaumont, Helen Tyrell and Stan Silverman (Buildings, Services and Funding);
- Olivia Williams, Emily Wolfe, Rachael Lee, David Eltringham (and Organisations and Sorting out NHS), Matthew Hopkins, Jason Stokes and Antony Townsend (Staff and Training);
- Oluwamayowa Olutobi (Organisations);
- Matthew Boissaud-Cooke and Kieren Caldwell (Specialists and Specialist Commissioning);
- Harmeet Kaur Harrar and Emma Fisher (Mental Health);
- Rogan Dean and Tessa Hewitt (Public Health);
- Angel Magar, Giovanni Bucci, Sonia Kandola, Kavi Sharma, Shivam Joshi, Tracy Gazeley, Natassia Garton and Nicolas Aldridge (Research);
- Thomas Dale MacLaine and Frances Griffiths (The Digital NHS);
- Sir Bruce Keogh, Professor Kiran Patel and Dame Stella Manzie MBE (Sorting out the NHS);
- Penny Kechagioglou (The Future of the NHS).

Yakup Kilic and James Korolewicz copy-edited and reviewed the whole book, and are a great inspiration to me. Aaron Ashmore helped me keep to a plan; and Abie Tutt, a dynamic final year medical student, gave me many great ideas.

I would especially like to thank Will Sloper, who combines being an ICU trainee doctor (quite busy through the pandemic), a father of two young children, doing anaesthetic exams, and designing the brilliant cartoons in each chapter. They make me laugh and I hope set the right tone for the book.

The publisher, Jonathan Wright, kept me to task and the project moving. Peter Ellis edited the book brilliantly, cutting it down from 120,000 to 70,000 words and making it readable. Sir Bruce Keogh (ex Medical Director of NHS England) both wrote a foreword, and gave an insight into the workings of NHS England, and added to the book. I thank them all. It would not have happened without them.

Foreword

The introduction to the NHS Constitution is clear:

> "The NHS belongs to the people. It is there to improve our health and wellbeing, supporting us to keep mentally and physically well, to get better when we are ill and, when we cannot fully recover, to stay as well as we can to the end of our lives. It works at the limits of science – bringing the highest levels of human knowledge and skill to save lives and improve health. It touches our lives at times of basic human need, when care and compassion are what matter most."

Our NHS arose after WW2, at a time of terrible hardship, to ensure that everybody - no matter who they were – could access the same healthcare, without ever having to worry about money or administrative hassle. This visionary product of bold democratic politics, based on the principle of pooling our individual risks of illness and national resources to meet our individual needs, became an icon of the British social conscience. But the pursuit of high-quality healthcare in the NHS requires continuous responsiveness to the unremitting and inter-related forces of emerging science and technology, relentlessly increasing demand, escalating costs, rising public expectations – and funding which is dependent on the success of the national economy.

The Coronavirus pandemic of 2020 has brought some of these considerations into sharp relief and rekindled an interest in the societal and economic value of NHS, that has not been seen since its inception in 1948. It has exposed the tension between medical, economic, social and political priorities in a cauldron of competing evidence and opinions.

This is why *Understanding the NHS* is so timely. It is not an academic thesis or a political treatise. It is a book for everyone with an interest in the NHS. Having set out the challenges and political and social context of the NHS over the last few decades, the authors make some proposals for "sorting out the NHS" in the future. Good people may agree or disagree with their proposals, or have alternative ideas. But to aspire to an NHS that is evidenced-based, focused on outcomes and patient-centred, change is constantly necessary – whether through national policy or local innovation.

To avoid change for the sake of change, all proposals should convincingly pass at least one of these seven tests. Will the proposed change:

1. Reduce demand by preventing disease or improving wellbeing?
2. Accelerate the time from seeking help to definitive treatment?
3. Enhance safety – before, during or after treatment?
4. Enable better clinical or health outcomes than at present?

5. Provide better taxpayer value?
6. Reduce inequality of access?
7. Improve the experience for patients?

These are the issues that matter. With all our health service's history, complexity, strengths and weaknesses, *Understanding the NHS* will inform debate and help us secure a brighter future for the NHS.

Professor Sir Bruce Keogh (National Medical Director, 2007-18)

Introduction

"People don't believe in ideas, they believe in people who believe in ideas"
Ze'ev Mankowitz

The NHS is more than a good idea. It is beautiful. And it is you. If you didn't believe in it, you probably would not be reading this book. And what an idea it is, one the greatest in modern compassionate society, i.e. to make healthcare equal. I hope this book enables you to do two things with that idea. One. Believe in it every day, and pass on that belief. Two. Work hard and lead the NHS throughout your career.

The idea, its beauty, and this book, have been in my head for most of my life. Why write it? I wanted to write down what I have learnt (and seen) over the last 60 years in the NHS. So how did it all start for me?

Well, I went to Nottingham Medical School in 1979 (it was newish, nine years old and felt 'fresh'). 1979 seems like anther age now. Industrial unrest helped Mrs Thatcher come to power. Devolution. Liverpool FC (my team) won the old 1st Division. Douglas Adams published his first masterpiece (as I saw it at the age of 17 years old), 'The Hitchhiker's Guide to the Galaxy'. In 1979, the NHS was still quite 'young' (31 years old). But my experience goes back to early childhood, in the early 60s – as I come from a medical family. And being the 7th Dr Stein (so far), I know, is not very original.

But not everyone has had my family's life story. My family's medical story starts post WW1. My maternal grandfather trained at the old Charing Cross Medical School (now part of Imperial College, London) and was a GP and Public Health Physician in Cheltenham in the 1920-30s. He met his wife, a nurse, as a junior doctor at Charing Cross Hospital. He was in the Army, went over in the British Expeditionary Force in WW1, was captured at Dunkirk and became a prisoner-of-war (ending up in Colditz) for 5 years - then a GP again. My mother trained at Newnham (Cambridge) and King's College London, which is now part of 'GKT' (Guys, Kings and Thomas'). She was an Obstetrician and Gynaecologist, then a GP, then a Public Health Physician, finishing her career as the Regional Medical Officer for SE Thames. Thus as a family, we have always had an interest in the 'bigger picture' (i.e. public health), not just the patient in front of us.

My father trained at Trinity College, Dublin, the first in his family to go to university. His father was a rag and bone man. My father was a GP, specialising in paediatrics, and a doctor in the RAF in WW2 - North Africa, Italy, the whole shebang. Post-war, as a GP before 1948, he established a practice in a poor area, in a poor town in Kent. He had a 'panel' (list) of patients but only working males were allowed on the list and received government-funded healthcare. Some were too poor to get on the list, and would pay him in kind, a farmer with eggs etc. Women and children were not a priority for the pre-NHS health system.

My parents worked together. Each would have alternate Thursday afternoons off and alternate weekends. Our home was the surgery. Opening my Dad's medical bag was never a good idea for a young child, usually leading to a question to him, "Where does this metal thing go? Does it hurt?". Contraceptive devices ended up in the cutlery drawer. You get the idea. So, we, as a family, lived and breathed the NHS, from before 1948, its birth and its history to date. I still do. That is a privilege.

But this book is for people who do not come from this background and do not have this life experience. They do not know how it works, and would like to know. They start off thinking it is one thing. Wrong. It is actually 7-8 silos that do not talk to each other. Each has different email and admin systems; different lines of finance; and different traditions, ambitions and ideas. They are also sometimes are in competition with each other. This makes people confused, frustrated and even angry, with the system. They do not know why it is so, and how to navigate themselves through the NHS.

Thus I have three target audiences. Firstly, I would like to educate health and social care students, and junior professionals in their early years; so they can start with my knowledge when I went to university in 1979. Secondly, it can contribute to career advice for 6th form students who are applying to university for a degree in health or social care. Thirdly, the book is for everyone else, who want to know how it all fits together; and in this way, improve their healthcare, and that of their family.

Thus, this book is written both for future and new health and social care professionals, and the interested general public. Its aim is to pass on the great idea, teach you how the NHS works, and enable you to provide better care for your patients, and receive better care (for you and your family).

Chapter 1

History of NHS: Beginning and Consolidation

This chapter describes the circumstances leading up to the establishment of the NHS, and its first 42 years and is an historical timeline with some medical context.

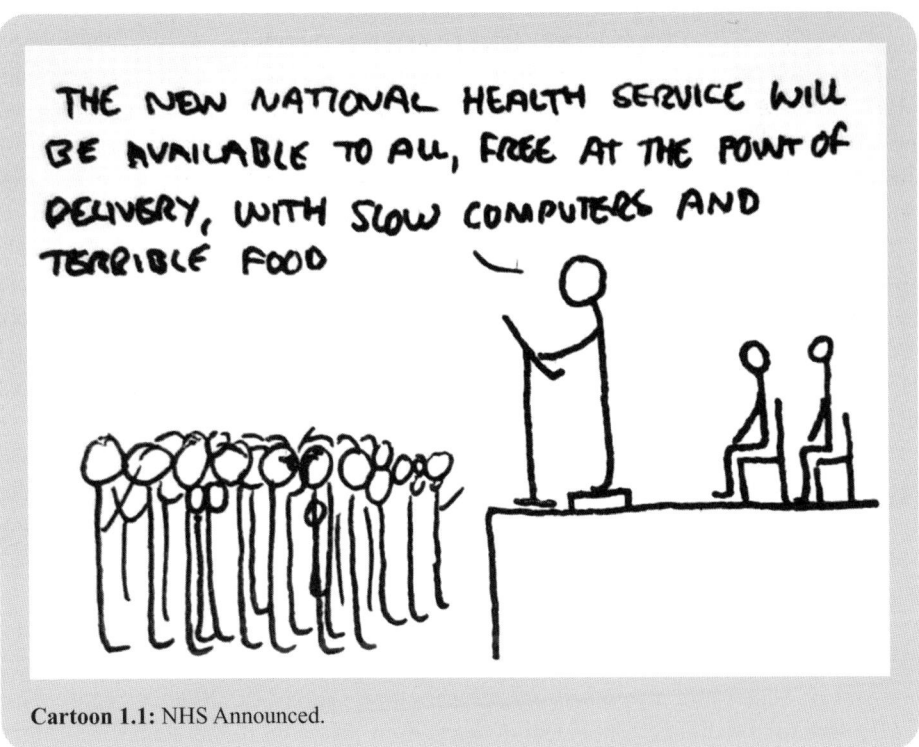

Cartoon 1.1: NHS Announced.

Introduction
Let's look at the word 'NHS'.

National: While the NHS covers all four constituent nations of the United Kingdom, it has taken different routes in each country. England and Wales have usually dovetailed, while Scotland and Northern Ireland exercise more autonomy.

Health: When the NHS was founded in 1948, male life expectancy at birth was 66 years. In 2020, it was 81. With this demographic transition comes an increased burden of chronic disease. Our ideas of health have similarly altered to include a more holistic account of health, supplementing physical fitness with mental, social, and spiritual wellbeing.

Service: What it means for the NHS to serve its public has changed over the course of its existence. Are the people sitting in the waiting room patients, clients, service users, or well-informed customers?

Pre-Twentieth Century Healthcare

In the 16th Century, the first Poor Law established almshouses to care for the poor and sick, with a system of 'outdoor relief'; providing benefits in kind to support the poor at home.

During the first half of the 19th Century, almshouses, and outdoor relief were thought to encourage dependency. So the State abolished direct welfare payments and established workhouses, austere large institutions for the care of the needy. Towards the end of the century, annexes were added to house the sick, the first *infirmaries*, in some respects, the first hospitals. Care was rudimentary with Florence Nightingale, amongst others, commenting on the atrocious conditions.

As the anatomical and pathological basis of disease became better understood, healthcare was increasingly provided by other bodies. Local councils established both 'Municipal Hospitals' for infectious diseases (many of which became 'District General Hospitals'), and institutions for people with mental or physical illnesses or intellectual disabilities.

Additionally, many 'Voluntary Hospitals' were established as charities where medical care was provided by visiting specialists who had lucrative private practice elsewhere. For economic reasons, such hospitals focused on people with acute problems not requiring long-term care. Some of these hospitals later became modern 'teaching hospitals' (see Chapter 6).

Primary and community care services evolved separately from the hospitals. Community care, including domiciliary, environmental and public health services, had always been the responsibility of the local authority. Regular epidemics, particularly of smallpox, typhus and cholera, drew attention to the need for sanitary and preventative measures. So from the mid-nineteenth century, local health boards had legal powers to protect water supplies, promote vaccination and enforce quarantines. However, it was not until the beginning of the twentieth century, that a primary care doctor service (i.e. a 'general practitioner', GP) was funded through insurance schemes.

This is the early timeline of healthcare development:
1808. **Mental Health.** County Asylums Act 1808 established *asylums* for poor and criminally insane, mentally ill people; the first opening in Northampton in 1811.

1815. **Apothecaries Act 1815** introduced compulsory apprenticeship and formal qualifications for apothecaries (later called general practitioners, GPs), under the license of the Society of Apothecaries.

1828. **Mental Health.** County Asylums Act 1828 required magistrates to send annual records of admissions, discharges, and deaths in asylums to the Home Office. It also imposed the requirement of a residential medical officer.

1832. **British Medical Association** launched under the name of the Provincial Medical and Surgical Association; with the objective of sharing medical knowledge.

1839. **Public Health.** The Poor Law Commission's fifth annual report. The report concluded the prevalence of disease was linked to substandard living conditions in England's industrial cities.

1841. **UK Census.** Estimated that a third of doctors in England were unqualified.

1845. **Mental Health.** Lunacy Act 1845 and County Asylums Act 1845. The Lunacy Acts changed the status of mentally ill people to patients.

1848. **Public Health.** Public Health Act 1848 and the General Board of Health established the General Board of Health and Local Boards, to advise on public health matters. The Act gave towns the right to appoint a Local Board of Health, led by a Medical Officer (now the Director of Public Health, DPH).

1853. **Public Health.** United Kingdom Vaccination Act 1853. Legislation made it compulsory for all children born after 1 August 1853 to be vaccinated against smallpox.

1854. **Public Health.** Improvements in Hospital Hygiene. Florence Nightingale returned from running military hospitals during the Crimean War, and instigated sanitary improvements in British hospitals, cementing the modern profession of nursing.

1858. **Medical Act 1858.** General Medical Council (GMC) was formed centralising the regulation of doctors in the UK.

1858. **Public Health.** Local Government Act 1858 abolished the General Board of Health. Its responsibilities were taken on by the Secretary of State for the Home Department, the Local Government Act Office, and the Privy Council.

1863. **Mental Health.** Establishment of first forensic mental health hospital in England, Broadmoor Criminal Lunatic Asylum.

1872 and 1875. **Public Health.** Further Public Health Acts enforced laws about slum clearance, provision of sewers and clean water.

1889-1902. **Public Health.** Arguably, discovering a third of those volunteering to fight in the Boer War (1899–1902) were rejected because of poor health, led the government to realise 'something had to be done' to improve the nation's health.

1890. **Mental Health.** Lunacy Act placed an obligation on local authorities to maintain institutions for the mentally ill.

Twentieth Century (pre-1940)

1905. **The Royal Commission on the Poor Law and the Unemployed.** The 'majority' and 'minority' reports released in 1909 criticised the duplication of health services provided by voluntary and Poor Law institutions, but their recommendations differed.

1910. **Origin of the phrase 'NHS'.** Dr Benjamin Moore was probably the first to use the words 'NHS' in *The Dawn of the Health Age*. He established the State Medical Service Association in 1912, replaced by the Socialist Medical Association in 1930.

1911. **National Insurance Act 1911.** Previously, systems of health insurance consisted of private schemes such as friendly societies or welfare societies. But in 1911, David Lloyd George (then Chancellor of the Exchequer) created a system whereby a small amount was deducted from weekly wages, supplemented by contributions from the employer.

Under this Act, all eligible working males could register with a GP. GPs who took part in this scheme were called 'panel doctors' and received an annual 'capitation' fee; a funding mechanism still used today. This was a very important act and in some ways, the real 'birth' of the NHS. For the first time, central government finance was used to provide medical care for the people.

1918. **Pandemic.** Spanish Flu (January 1918 - December 1920). Was caused by the transmission of an avian influenza virus to humans killing about 50 million people worldwide. It was followed by similar viral pandemics including Asian Flu (1957; 2 million deaths), Hong Kong Flu (1968; 1 million), HIV/AIDS (1981+, 33 million+), Swine Flu (2009; 300,000), Ebola (2013; 11,000) and COVID-19 (2020; over 5 million in November 2021).

1919. **Ministry of Health.** The First World War was a catalyst for social change with Lloyd George promising a land "fit for heroes to live in". This included the creation of the Ministry of Health.

1919. **Nurses Registration Act 1919.** This established a regulator for nurses, the General Nursing Council for England and Wales.

1920. **Dawson Report** suggested the organisation of medicine was insufficient to bring the advances of medical knowledge within the reach of the people.

1924. **Royal Commission on National Health Insurance.** The Commission's 'majority report', in 1926, found the system effective and recommended its extension to dependents. Its 'minority report' found the involvement of industrial insurance companies detrimental to the expansion of public health and recommended provision through public funding.

1929. **Local Government Act** allowed local authorities to run services over and above those authorised by the Poor Laws.

1930. **Socialist Medical Association** formed, and in his first Presidential address in May 1931, Somerville Hastings (a Labour politician and surgeon) outlined the principles for a new type of medical service: *preventive, universal and without economic barriers.*

1934. **Labour Conference (Southport).** The party ratified a motion on the creation of an NHS by Somerville Hastings.

1938. The British Medical Association (BMA) published a pamphlet: **'A General Medical Service for the Nation'**. It described how health insurance should be extended to the dependents of wage-earners.

The 1940s

1939. At the outbreak of war, central government took over voluntary and municipal hospitals establishing the **Emergency Medical Service**. Doctors and nurses were, for the first time, employed by a centralised state-run system. Oddly, healthcare often advances in war.

1942. An Inter-Departmental Committee led by Sir William Beveridge published the **Beveridge Report** calling for a comprehensive system of social insurance 'from cradle to grave'. It proposed all working people should pay a weekly contribution to the State with benefits to be paid to the unemployed, the sick, the retired, and the widowed. This is one of the most important documents in the social history of the UK and might be considered the manifesto of the *Welfare State*.

1946 (July). **NHS Act 1946** published.

1948. **Creation of the NHS.**

Following WWII, Britain's first majority Labour government, led by Clement Attlee, formulated plans for a comprehensive Welfare State. A *free at point-of-delivery* NHS was the cornerstone of these plans.[1]

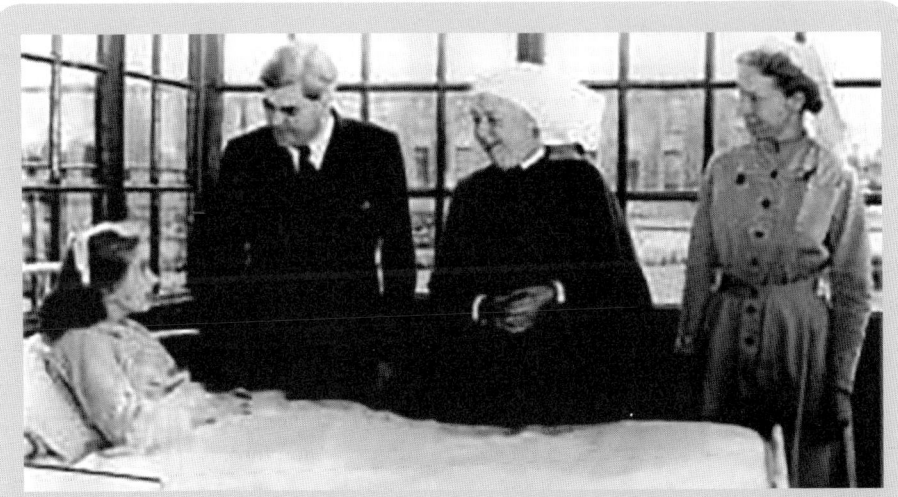

Picture 1.1: Aneurin Bevan, Minister of Health, on the first day of the National Health Service, 5 July 1948, at Park Hospital, Davyhulme, near Manchester.

---

1. It nearly did not happen. Famously, the BMA voted against it just before its birth. A Polish Diamond Merchant called Max Ryba identified Jewish and East European doctors who talked around many GPs.

The chief architect of the NHS was Labour Minister of Health, Aneurin Bevan. On 5 July, he launched the NHS at Park Hospital in Manchester (Trafford General Hospital).

The NHS in Scotland and Northern Ireland were legally distinct from England from the beginning, Wales, however, was managed from England and treated much like an English region for the first 20 years. This is what the 'tripartite system' of the new NHS looked like in 1948.

Hospitals
- State owned (nationalised) hospitals. 1.143 voluntary and 1,545 municipal hospitals became the responsibility of 14 Regional Hospital Boards in England and Wales.
- The 36 'Teaching Hospitals' had different arrangements and were organised under Boards of Governors. Hospital consultants retained the right to conduct their private practice as well as gaining full-time salaried employment in the NHS. This is still the case.
- In 1948 hospitals were managed by a medical superintendent, a matron and a lay administrator (called the 'secretary')[2].

General practice
- The national network of general practitioners extended (and replaced) the 'panel system' and included the entire population. GPs were responsible for primary

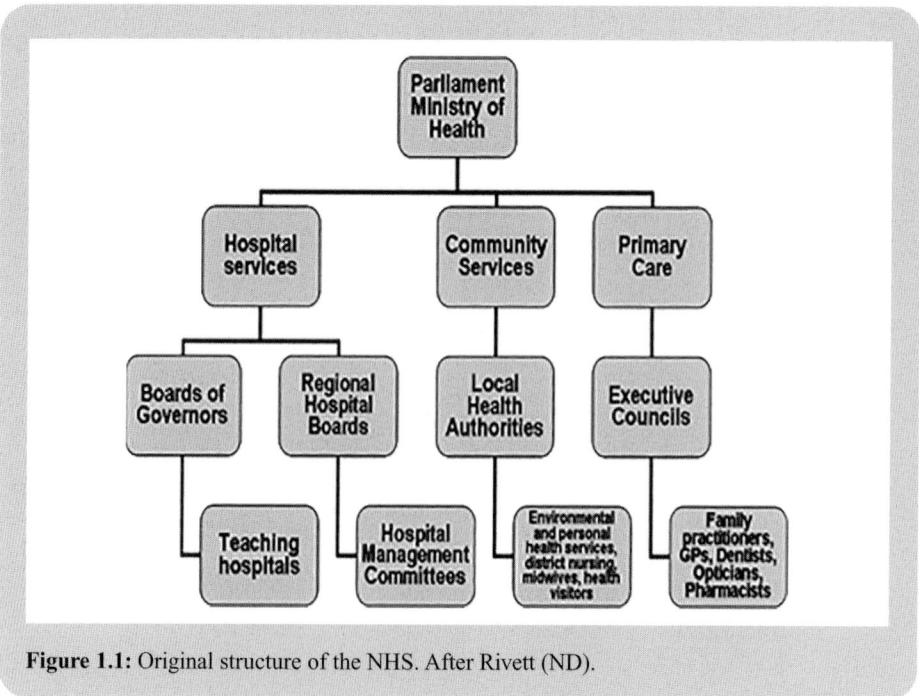

Figure 1.1: Original structure of the NHS. After Rivett (ND).

---

2. AS's mother was a junior doctor post-war and reminds him that, in large London hospitals she worked in, the 'hospital secretary' was the only administrator. We now have many 100s per hospital.

healthcare and received fees which were set and paid nationally. Each person would be registered to a specific GP. On 5 July 1948 (when the NHS officially 'started'), 86% of all GPs joined it, and over the next six months the proportion rose to 96%.

Community and domiciliary health services
- Maternity and child welfare clinics, health visitors, midwives, health education, ambulance services, public and environmental health and health promotion (including vaccination) continued to be run by City or County councils (Local Authorities), which were also responsible for housing, roads and education.

The NHS's original management structures in 1948 consisted of:
- 14 Regional Health Boards (RHBs)
- 36 boards of governors for teaching hospitals (BGs)
- 388 hospital management committees (HMCs)
- 138 executive councils (ECs)
- 147 local health authorities (LHAs).

The NHS made an immediate impact on the health and imagination of the nation. In 1952, Aneurin Bevan said:

"The essence of a satisfactory health service is that the rich and the poor are treated alike, that poverty is not a disability, and wealth is not advantaged."

The strands of the tripartite system had, and still have, different funding streams and were managed separately. This was possibly the biggest mistake in the NHS – made at its creation.

The Central Health Services Council (CHSC) was created by the 1946 NHS Act and was the advisory mechanism for the Ministry of Health. It had substantial representation from the professions as well as members from local government and hospital management.

There were also Standing Advisory Committees which remained in existence until 2005: the Standing Medical Advisory Committee (SMAC); Standing Nursing and Midwifery Advisory Committee (SNMAC), Standing Pharmaceutical services Advisory Committee (SPAC) and Standing Dentistry Advisory Committee (SDAC).

Even though the NHS 'started' in 1948, we hope you can see, it was really a development of previous organisations and Acts of Parliament. This gathered pace from the start of the Twentieth Century and the National Insurance Act of 1911 was vital. Its formation was beautiful (in our eyes)[3].

1948. **Health Services Act (Northern Ireland) 1948.**

1949. The **Nurses Act 1949** established a framework for the role of nursing within the NHS.

---

3. The concept was (and is) both an intrinsic part of a fair society, and brilliant and beautiful, in our view. We should all be proud of the NHS. And, we all have a duty to protect and develop it.

1949. The **NHS (Amendment) Act 1949** safeguarded the independence of GPs. It also proposed prescription charges of not more than one shilling per prescription. However, due to intense opposition, the charges were not implemented until 1952.

The 1950s
After initial success in the eyes of the public, costs started to spiral. So various services were then taken out of the new NHS. Mass vaccination and intensive care started. First Clean Air and Mental Health Acts.

1950. **Education**. Medical Act 1950 introduced disciplinary boards and a compulsory year of training for doctors after their university qualification.

1950. **Research.** First UK Report Linking Smoking to Lung Cancer.

1952. **Prescriptions, Dental charges (mainly dentures) and Spectacles.** Originally 'free', charges for these items were now introduced. As of 2021 prescription charges remain in England, but were abolished in Wales, Northern Ireland and Scotland in 2007, 2010 and 2011.

1952. **Royal College of General Practice** established.

1952. **Clinical.** Birth of Intensive Care Concept.

1953. **Research.** Structure of Deoxyribonucleic Acid (DNA) described.

1955. **Clinical.** UK's First Kidney Transplant.

1956. **Public Health.** The Clean Air Act was a response to worsening air pollution in urban areas of the UK; the 1952 *Great Smog* in London killing an estimated 12,000 people.

First Mass Vaccination Programme. Polio and diphtheria jabs were offered to under fifteens.

1959. **Clinical.** First General ICUs in UK.

1959. **Mental Health Act** recommended, where possible, treatment in the community - and mental and physical health should have equal status.

The 1960s
Oral contraception, and the Abortion Act, contribute to the changing roles of men and women in society.

1961. **Public Health.** Oral Contraceptive Pill. The contraceptive pill gave women birth control, though only available to married women until 1967.

1962. **Birth of the Modern Hospital.** A "Hospital Plan for England and Wales" was proposed by Health Minister, Enoch Powell, as a ten-year vision for hospital building. 14 Regional Health Boards (RHBs) oversaw planning and building of one new DGH per 125,000 of population. This led to 90 new hospitals, with 134 extensively remodelled.

All DGHs were to have Accident and Emergency and Outpatient Departments. Single-speciality hospitals went out of favour, except in London, where single organ hospitals (like the Moorfield Eye Hospital) still exist. Only people requiring specialised care, e.g. cardiac and neurosurgery, needed to travel to regional teaching hospitals, which were mostly in big cities.

1962. **Medical Services Review Committee's final report (Porritt Report)** proposed a reform of the tripartite system, with the administration and co-ordination of medical and other services, under one Area Health Authority.

1964. **Artificial Fluoridation of Water Supply.**

1964. **Clinical.** First Coronary Care Unit (CCU) in UK (Edinburgh).

1967. **Public Health.** NHS Family Planning and Abortion Acts made abortion legal up to 28 weeks (24 weeks in 1990) if a woman's mental or physical health was at risk. The Act did not cover Northern Ireland until 2020.

1967. **Research.** Whitehall Studies (large prospective cohort studies) commenced, investigating social determinants of health - specifically the cardiovascular disease prevalence and mortality rates among British civil servants.

1967. **Salmon Committee's Report (Senior Nursing Staff Structure)** made recommendations for developing staff structure and embedding the profession in hospital management - heralding the end of the traditional matron.

1967. **Joint Working Party on the Organisation of Medical Work, First (Cogwheel) Report** encouraged the involvement of clinicians in management and proposed specialty groupings, e.g. medical and surgical divisions.

1968. **Public Health.** Clean Air Act (Second) introduced measures to reduce air pollution.

1968. **Department of Health and Social Security (DHSS).** The Ministry of Health was dissolved, and its functions transferred (with the Ministry of Social Security) to the new DHSS. Twenty years later, these functions were split into: the Department of Social Security (DSS) and the Department of Health (DH), renamed the Department of Health and Social Care (DHSC) in 2018.

1968. **Pandemic.** Hong Kong Flu. The H3N2 influenza virus spread across the world, lasting until 1972; it killed approximately one million people.

1968. **Clinical.** UK's First Liver Transplant.

1968. **Clinical.** UK's First Heart Transplant.

1968. **Committee on Local Authority and Allied Social Services' Report** advised an amalgamation of welfare services, home help, mental health and social work services to create a unified social services department.

1969. **Responsibility for the NHS in Wales** was passed to the Secretary of State for Wales. The NHS in Scotland and Northern Ireland had developed separately from 1948.

The 1970s
Major re-organisation of the NHS (1974). GPs started a mandatory three-year training.

1970. **Local Authority Social Services Act** carried through the recommendations of the Seebohm Report, creating a single social service department in every local authority.

1971. **Technology.** First Computerised Tomography (CT) Scan in UK.

1972. **Royal College of General Practitioners** given royal charter.

1972. **Public Health.** Faculty of Public Health created as standard setting body.

1973. **Clinical.** First Successful Bone Marrow Transplant in a child in the UK.

1974. **NHS Reorganisation (Major) Act 1973** was the biggest reorganisation of the NHS in its history; abolishing the 14 RHBs, HMCs, and most teaching hospital boards (except those of the London postgraduate teaching hospitals).

The 14 RHBs, with minor boundary changes, became Regional Health Authorities (RHAs) with a focus on strategic planning. Operational authority was delegated to 90 new Area Health Authorities (AHAs), assisted by Family Practitioner Committees (FPCs) and Community Health Councils (CHCs); all coterminous with one local authority. The AHAs in turn supervised 192 District Health Authorities (DHAs).

Joint Consultative Committees were created between the NHS and Local Authorities, the latter providing social services, housing and education. These tried to bridge the gaps between the three domains of the original 'tripartite system'.

FPCs were created with responsibility for GP, dental, pharmaceutical and ophthalmic services. FPCs were abolished in 1990 and replaced by family health services authorities.

CHCs were created in each AHA to provide a voice for patients and the public in the NHS in England and Wales. Their work is now done by Healthwatch England.

Local authorities retained responsibility for public health measures related to food hygiene and environmental health, but preventive medical issues become the responsibility of the NHS (returned to local government in 2013).

The Health Service Ombudsman was created - later the Health Service Commissioner of England, Scotland and Wales. The Health Service Commissioner for England still retains the post of Parliamentary Commissioner for Administration - now more commonly called the Parliamentary and Health Service Ombudsman (PHSO).

1974. **NHS Reorganisation in Northern Ireland.** Hospitals, managed by the Northern Ireland Hospitals Authority and Hospital Management Committees from 1948 to 1974, were transferred to four integrated health and social services boards.

1975. **Public Health.** Resource Allocation Working Party (RAWP)[4] was established to distribute health funding more fairly across the UK.

---

4. AS's mother was Regional Medical Officer of SE Thames (one of the 4 London regions of the time) and involved with RAWP. She thought it was a 'good thing' despite taking investment away from London.

RAWP suggested using Standardised Mortality Ratios as a proxy for calculating regional burdens of disease. The formula devised by RAWP survived until 1989, reducing the funding gap between the Northern regions and London. It was replaced by a more complex formula announced in the publication of 'Working for Patients' in 1989. There have since been further changes and debate, particularly about the relative weighting for old age which favoured the more prosperous South; whereas a model based on relative deprivation favours the North.

1978. **Clinical.** World's First Test Tube Baby. On 25 July, the world's first 'test tube baby' was born.

1978. **Research.** Last Case of Smallpox in the World. The only virus eradicated from humanity through our actions.

1979. **Nurses, Midwives and Health Visitors Act 1979.**

The 1980s

Black Report confirmed inequalities according to socio-economic status. HIV/AIDS spread around the world. 1989 White Paper 'Working for Patients' heralded the Internal Market.

1980. **Public Health.** The Black Report commissioned by Labour (in 1977) showed inequalities existed in access to health services, and mortality, between social groups and the gap was widening.

1980. **Technology.** First Magnetic Resonance Imaging (MRI) in UK.

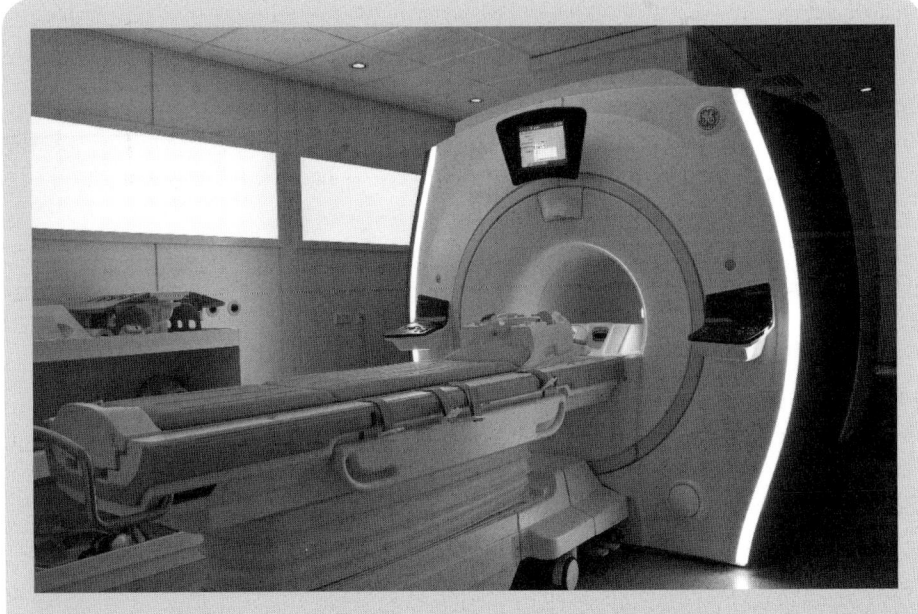

Pic 1.2: MRI machine.

1981. **Pandemic.** HIV/AIDS. First AIDs Cases reported in USA.

1982. **NHS Reorganisation (Minor).** The first Thatcher government considered excess bureaucracy had been created by the 1974 reforms and removed AHAs.

1983. **Public Health.** Seat belt use made compulsory in the UK.

1983. **Mental Health.** (Second) Mental Health Act 1983 introduced the issue of consent and set out when people can be detained, or 'sectioned'.

1983. **Griffiths Report** ushered in a more business-like model in NHS management; with professional, well paid, general managers taking over cost control; and clinical and professional staff (except medical and surgical consultants) becoming responsible to managers.

The Health Services Supervisory Board (HSSB) was created to set policy. It was chaired by the Secretary of State but removed him/her from day-to-day involvement. This morphed into the NHS Management Board in 1985. This board, in turn, became the NHS Executive in 1996 and was disbanded in 2002 to form four Regional Directorates of Health and Social Care (themselves abolished in 2003, with functions absorbed back into the Department of Health).

1983. **Medical Act 1983** provided the current statutory basis for the General Medical Council's functions.

1983. **United Kingdom Central Council (UKCC) for Nursing, Midwifery and Health Visiting** replaced the General Nursing Council for England and Wales, the Central Midwives Board and seven other bodies.

1986. **Epidemic.** 'Mad Cow Disease'. Bovine spongiform encephalopathy (BSE) affected cows in the UK in the 1980s and 1990s. A variant crossed into humans.

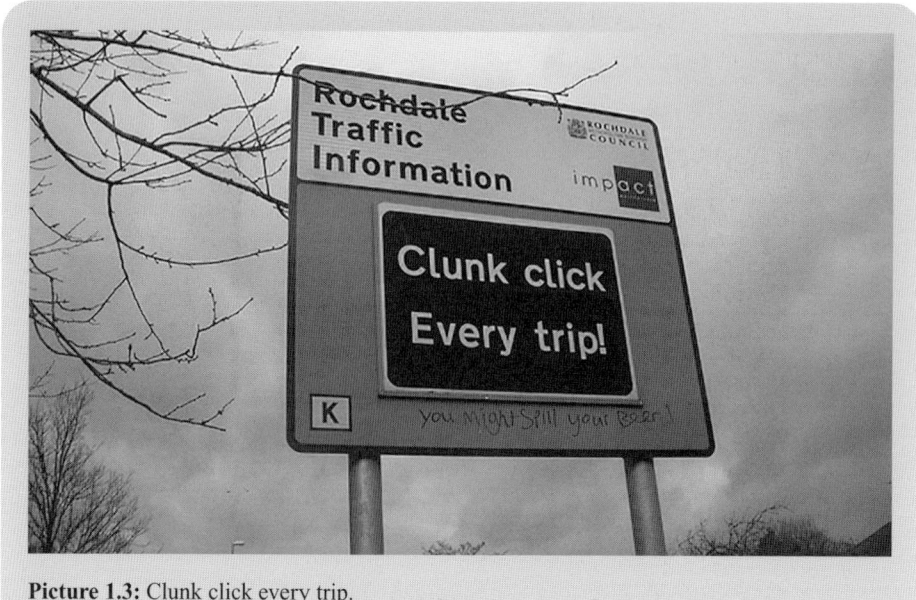

Picture 1.3: Clunk click every trip.

1986. **Public Health.** First AIDS Health Campaign: 'AIDS: Don't Die of Ignorance' to raise awareness of HIV.

1986. **Clinical.** Cardiac Thrombolysis. A study, published in *The Lancet,* was the first to demonstrate the efficacy of cardiac thrombolysis (streptokinase) in acute myocardial infarction.

1987. **Clinical.** World's First Heart, Lung and Liver transplant.

1987. **'Promoting Better Health'** government white paper focused on health promotion and prevention reforms. The government reviewed payments systems for GPs to encourage efficiency and boost preventive medicine, leading to changes in the GP contract in 1990.

1988. **Public Health.** Breast and Cervical Cancer Screening. Mammograms introduced for women aged over 50, and cervical cancer screening for women aged 20 to 64 years.

1989. **'Working for Patients'** government white paper introduced an 'internal market' to the NHS, including:
- An introduction of an 'internal market' through the separation of 'providers' (e.g. hospitals) and 'purchasers' (commissioning or buying healthcare)
- The establishment of independent (later Foundation) 'Trusts', directly accountable to government
- The creation of 'fund-holding GPs' enabling them to buy hospital services directly (mainly outpatient services, elective operations, care and diagnostic procedures)
- The use of non-legal 'contracts' for payment for services between purchasers and providers
- The change to a capitation (weighted population) basis ('tariff') for purchasing services for a given population; in place of direct funding of services
- Introduction of capital charges for buildings/equipment
- The promotion of medical audit and job plans for consultants.

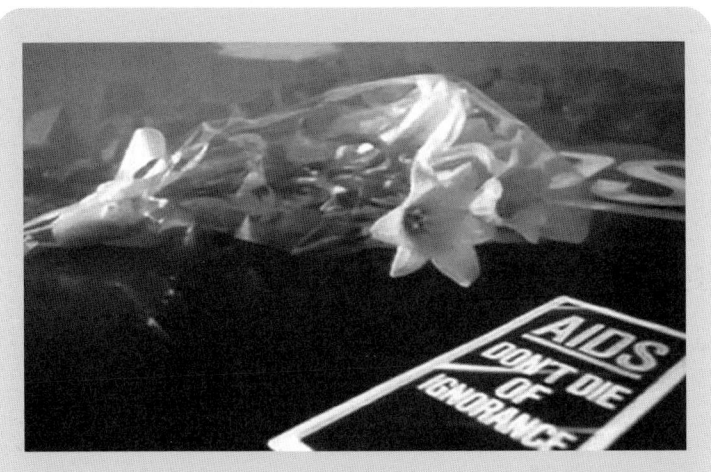

Picture 1.4: AIDS: don't die of ignorance.

Chapter 2

History of NHS: Modernisation

This chapter continues the history of the NHS, from 1990 onwards. This was a key turning point with the advent of the 'internal market'.

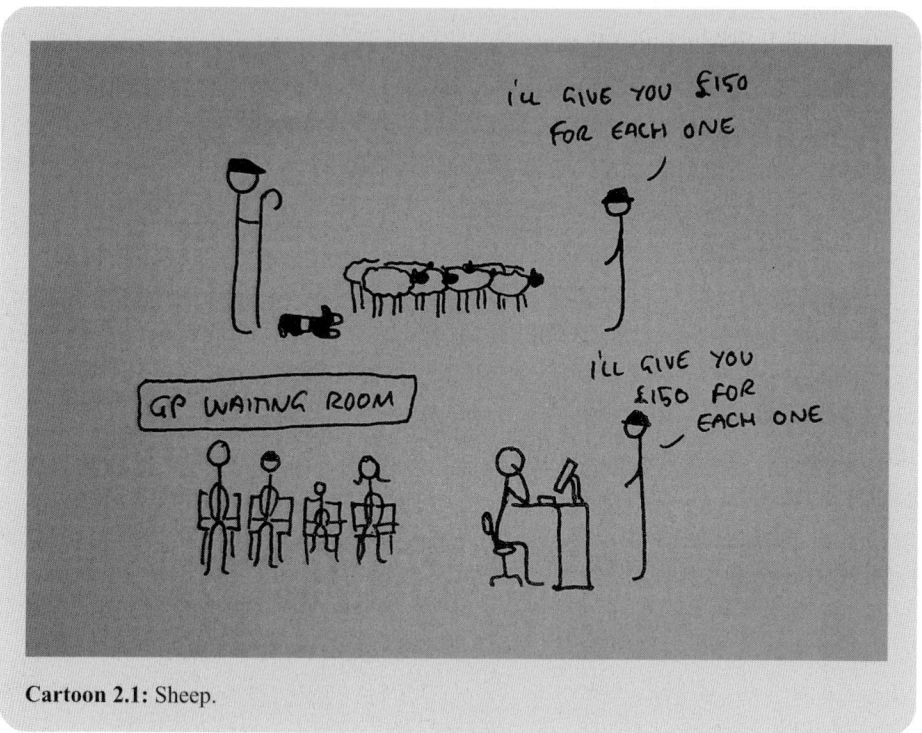

Cartoon 2.1: Sheep.

Introduction

By 1990, the foundations of the modern NHS were in place. There was a structure, with local commissioning organisations (made up of GPs and lay representatives), purchasing the services of secondary and tertiary care centres. There was only one major restructuring in the first forty years of the NHS. But in the last thirty, there has been an acceleration, with complex reorganisations instituted in 1990, 1995, 2001, 2013 and 'now' (2021-2).

Important performance markers ('targets') were devised, along with regulatory organisations, such as the CQC, NICE and Dr Foster. All of this may have made the NHS more efficient (and safer) but also more complex.

The 1990s
A lot happened in the 90s. This includes the introduction of:
- The 'Internal Market' (introducing 'purchasers', 'providers' and 'GP fund-holders')
- Independent hospital 'Trusts'
- The Patient's Charter (suggesting 'targets')
- A focus on junior doctors' hours
- Percutaneous Coronary Interventions (PCIs)
- Organ donor register
- Minor Injuries Units
- Stroke Thrombolysis
- Further NHS Re-organisation
- National Institute for Clinical Excellence – later National Institute for Health and Care Excellence (NICE)
- NHS Direct
- Primary Care Groups
- Commission for Health Improvement
- National IT strategy
- National Service Frameworks.

1990. **NHS Reorganisation (Major).** NHS and Community Care Act 1990. Introduced the 'NHS internal market', with District Health Authorities (DHAs) acting as 'purchasers' with their own budgets, buying care from hospitals ('providers'). Hospitals could apply for trust status. General practices were given 'fundholding budgets' subtracted from the host DHA's budget.

1990. **Human Fertility and Embryology Act 1990** created the Human Fertilisation and Embryology Authority.

1990. **GP Contract Changes.** Following proposals in the 1987 White Paper 'Promoting Better Health', the new contract incentivised GPs through performance-related payments. Following negotiation, the Secretary of State allowed seniority payments to remain, but GPs did not welcome the new arrangements.

1990. **Public Health.** Food Safety Act 1990. Made it a statutory obligation to treat food intended for human consumption in a controlled way.

1990. **Technology.** First Laparoscopic Cholecystectomy in UK.

1991. **First NHS Trusts.** As part of the internal market, hospitals could apply for 'trust status', giving them more financial and governance independence. 57 NHS trusts were established on 1 April 1991 under the NHS and Community Care Act 1990.

1991. **Junior Doctors Hours.** The Government announced no junior doctor should be working more than 83 hours a week by the following April[5]. The UK and European

---

5. AS's mother, a doctor, reminded him at the time that 'in her day' junior doctors had no truly free 'time off', unless sanctioned by their consultant. This allowed for wedding days and not much else.

averages at the time were 89 and 59 hours, respectively. Their working hours were limited by law in 2004 to 58 hours a week; and then, by 2009, to 48 hours.

1991. **Health of the Nation (HoN) White Paper and Patient's Charter.** The report highlighted the responsibilities of health authorities to concentrate on cost-effective strategies for dealing with major causes of ill-health; and emphasised the actions that individuals could take to safeguard their own health.

The report led to a Patient's Charter which set out the rights of patients in the NHS. It was revised in 1995 and 1997, before evolving into the NHS Constitution in 2009. Broad targets were set for the improvement of health in the nation to be achieved within four years, including: reduced waiting times for an emergency ambulance (14 mins for urban areas, and 19 mins in rural districts); 5 minute wait in A&E; limited cancellation of operations; named nurses, named midwives and health visitors responsible for patients' care; arrangements for discharge from hospital; waiting times for out-patients (30 minutes to be seen, and no more than two years for treatment).

1992. **Research.** UK Cochrane Collaboration. This international network was established to prepare, maintain and disseminate systematic reviews of research on the effects of healthcare - as part of a drive towards evidence-based medicine.

1992. **Tomlinson Review** recommended the merger of Guy's and Thomas' hospitals and the closure of Charing Cross, Middlesex, and St Bartholomew's alongside ten smaller hospitals. The government accepted the report. While Middlesex closed, and Guy's and Thomas' did merge, most of the recommendations were not implemented because they were too controversial.

1993. **Calman Report** reduced the minimum length of consultant training to seven years and introduced explicit curricula leading to a 'Certificate of Completion of Specialist Training' (CCST). After this, a UK doctor could be added to the GMC's 'Specialist Register' and apply for consultant posts. 'Registrar' and 'Senior Registrar (or 'SR')'[6] (middle stage of training) grades were merged into the Specialist Registrar ('SpR') training grade, and later the Speciality Trainee ('ST') grade.

1993. **Public Health.** Clean Air Act 1993. This dealt with issues such as height of chimneys on trade and industrial premises and the use of authorised fuels.

1993. **Technology.** Percutaneous Coronary Intervention (PCI) / Stents.

1994. **Public Health.** Organ Donor Register.

1994. **Clinical.** First Nurse-led Minor Injuries Unit.

1995. **Research.** Stroke Thrombolysis.

1995. **NHS Reorganisation (Major).** Health Authorities Act 1995. The fourteen regional health authorities (RHAs) were abolished and replaced in 1996 by the 'NHS Executive', and its eight regional offices. The 192 DHAs were replaced by 95 larger 'Health Authorities'.

---

6. AS was the last 'renal SR' in South London.

1997. **Public Health.** First Minister of Public Health. The post had disappeared by the time of the COVID-19 (C19) - which probably contributed to our poor performance.

1997. **'The New NHS: Modern, Dependable'** government white paper. The purchaser/provider split continued, with 'purchasing' rebranded as 'commissioning'. It also proposed publishing comparative information on NHS trust performance, which evolved into 'targets', e.g. the 4-hour A&E wait - drawing categories from the Patient's Charter.

1997. **Avian Flu outbreak.** An outbreak of Influenza A virus subtype H5N1 occurred in Hong Kong. Another outbreak of a different variant (Influenza A virus subtype H7N9) occurred in 2013, with a higher mortality.

1998. **Public Health.** Independent Inquiry into Inequalities in Health Report (Acheson Report) found that despite an overall downward trend in mortality from 1970–1990, the upper social classes experienced a more rapid improvement.

1998. **Information Technology.** NHS Direct. A telephone service for non-emergency health problems was rolled out across England in 2000, followed by Wales in 2001; replaced in 2013 by 'NHS 111' in England, Wales and Scotland.

1999. **Public Health.** 'Saving Lives: Our Healthier Nation' white paper set a national target of 300,000 lives saved over the next decade with a specific focus on: cancer, coronary heart disease and stroke, accidents, and mental illness.

1999. **Public Health.** National Institute for Clinical Excellence (NICE). Created to serve the English and Welsh NHS, NICE is an independent organisation providing national guidance on health promotion and the prevention and treatment of illness.

1999. **NHS Reorganisation (Minor).** Health Act 1999. Formally abolished GP fundholding and made provision for the establishment of primary care trusts (PCTs, which would evolve from primary care groups, PCGs).

The Commission for Health Improvement (CHI) was formed as the first organisation to assess the clinical performance of NHS hospitals. It was subsumed by the Healthcare Commission in 2001, which became the Care Quality Commission (CQC) in 2009.

1999. **Information Technology.** NHS Information Authority (NHSIA) (Establishment and Constitution) Order 1999 brought together four NHS IT and Information bodies in England. It became part of Health and Social Care Information Centre (HSCIC) in 2005.

1999. **Public Health.** Food Standards Agency Act 1999.

1999. **National Service Frameworks (NSFs).** These 10-year plans for chronic conditions which included an NSF were issued for mental health in 1999, and for coronary heart disease in 2000. Experienced clinicians advised the Chief Medical Officer (CMO), becoming Health Directors, or 'tsars', driving clinical policies for cancer, heart disease, mental health, and older people's services. Three of the Standing Committees were abolished in 2005, and one (dental) in 2010. NSFs were discontinued in 2013.

The 2000s
A lot happened in this decade as well:
- Internal market adapted
- NHS Plan, and targets were introduced, and some services outsourced to the private sector
- Walk-in Centres
- Dr Foster
- PCGs become PCTs
- SARS-Coronavirus
- Foundation Trusts (encouraging financial independence)
- Bristol, Shipman and Alder Hey scandals
- GPs partly paid by QoF points
- Emphasis on mental health with Mental Care Act (MCA) and IAPTs
- 'Choice' agenda
- CHI/Healthcare Commission/CQC
- NHS Constitution.

The congestion charge and the smoking ban were arguably the most influential measures.

2000. **The NHS Plan: A plan for investment. A plan for reform.** The ten-year plan for the NHS in England combined a commitment to substantial investment with radical changes. The most controversial aspects of the plan were a major Private Finance Initiative (PFI) hospital building programme; and the introduction of more private sector providers, cementing the competitive internal market.

The plan stated that:

"by 2004 no-one should be waiting more than four hours in accident and emergency from arrival to admission, transfer or discharge".

It has not been achieved since July 2015.

There was also a focus on elective care (operations, etc). In 2004 this crystallised into the ambition to reduce waiting times from '18 months to 18 weeks'. By December 2008, waiting times for elective care had fallen substantially: 90.3% of admitted and 96.8% of non-admitted patients were seen within 18 weeks. In October 2021, it is 65.6% in England.

2000. **10-year NHS Cancer Plan and Two-Week Cancer Target.** Following the introduction in 1999 of a maximum two week wait for a specialist appointment for cases of suspected breast cancer, the Cancer Plan announced this would be rolled out for all cancers by December 2000 - now a right under the NHS Constitution. The plan built on existing cancer initiatives, providing a comprehensive strategy across the whole patient pathway, establishing 34 local cancer networks in England.

2000. **Clinical.** NHS 'Walk-in Centres'. In April 1999, DH authorised funding for a pilot scheme of 40 NHS walk-in centres in England, the first of which opened in London in January 2000.

2000. **Public Health.** Health Development Agency (HDA). Following its announcement in the 1999 'Saving Lives: our Healthier Nation' White Paper, the Health Development Agency (HDA) was created as a successor 'special health authority' to the Health Education Council (1969-1987) and the Health Education Authority (1987-2000). Its purpose was to develop an evidence base to improve health and reduce health inequalities in partnership across a range of sectors. The functions of the HDA were transferred to NICE in 2005.

2000. **Information Technology.** The Dr Foster unit started at Imperial College (London) monitoring the performance of the NHS and providing information to the public.

2001. **NHS Reorganisation (Major).** Health and Social Care Bill 2001. Primary Care Trusts (PCTs) started forming out of Primary Care Groups (PCGs) with the remit of commissioning primary, community and secondary health services. Collectively the 303 PCTs spent around 80 per cent of the NHS budget. They were abolished in April 2013 as part of the Health and Social Care (HSC) Act 2012, being replaced by Clinical Commissioning Groups (CCGs). The 95 Health Authorities became 28 Strategic Health Authorities (SHAs) with a sub-regional role.

2001. **Public Health.** The Health Select Committee Report on Public Health found blurred lines of responsibility between health and local government.

2001. **Public Health.** The Food Standards Agency (FSA) was created taking responsibility for food hygiene and nutritional policy.

2001. **Nursing and Midwifery Order 2001** established the Nursing and Midwifery Council as the nursing and midwifery regulator, taking over from the UKCC.

2001. **Scandal.** The Bristol Inquiry chaired by Professor Ian Kennedy QC concluded the Bristol Royal Infirmary were 'simply not up to the task' because of shortages of surgeons and nurses, and a lack of leadership, accountability, and teamwork.

2002. **NHS Reorganisation (Minor).** The NHS Executive was divided into 4 Regional Directorates, themselves abolished in 2003; as the 28 SHAs (formed in 2001) had taken over the sub-regional remit.

2002. **Epidemic.** Severe Acute Respiratory Syndrome Coronavirus (SARS-CoV) outbreak. Thought to have originated from bats and spread to other animals (civet cats). There were 774 deaths. This was not bad enough to herald what was to come with C19.

2002. **Public Health.** The 'Getting ahead of the curve - A strategy for combating infectious diseases' strategy document proposed to establish a new National Infection Control and Health Protection Agency (the latter was formed in 2004).

2002. **Foundation Trust** system, was announced to liberate the best hospitals from central governmental control and encourage them to compete to provide better care.

2002. **Scandal.** The Shipman Inquiry reported on the serial killer and GP Harold Shipman. Shipman was found guilty of 15 murders in January 2000 (later thought to be approximately

250 murders). It led to the GMC creating a compulsory yearly 'appraisal' and 5 yearly 'revalidations' for all senior doctors in the UK.

2003. **Community Health Councils** abolished, as part of the NHS Plan 2000; and were replaced, in England, by Public and Patient Involvement Forums, subsequently replaced by local involvement networks (LINks), themselves superseded by Healthwatch England in 2013.

2003. **Public Health.** The Medicines and Healthcare products Regulatory Agency (MHRA) established, from a merger of the Medicines Control Agency (MCA) and the Medical Devices Agency (MDA); responsible for ensuring medicines and medical devices work and are acceptably safe. In April 2013, the MHRA merged with the National Institute for Biological Standards and Control (NIBSC) which became a 'centre' within it.

2003. **Public Health.** The '5-a-day' Campaign was launched to encourage people to eat more fruit and vegetables.

2003. **Public Health.** Focus on Homelessness. The 2002 Rough Sleepers Unit target to reduce the number of people sleeping rough by two-thirds was met a year earlier than planned.

2003. **Physician Associates.** PAs, medically trained generalist healthcare professionals, who work alongside doctors under defined levels of supervision, were formally introduced to the NHS. PAs are currently regulated by the Faculty of Physician Associates with the GMC expected to take on regulation from late 2021.

2004. **Four-Hour A&E Target** started. It was, and remains, the primary performance indicator for emergency care in the NHS, being modified from 100% to 98% in 2004 to allow 'clinical exceptions', e.g. patients undergoing active resuscitation. The target was reduced to 95% in 2010.

2004. **18 Week Referral to Treatment (RTT) Target** commenced and remains the primary performance indicator for planned care.

2004. **Public Health.** The Healthcare Commission, with the legal name of 'The Commission for Healthcare Audit and Inspection' (CHAI), was created by a parliamentary act in 2003, and took over the role of the Commission for Health Improvement (CHI) in 2004. It also assumed some of the responsibilities of the National Care Standards Commission (NCSC) and the Audit Commission. The Commission was abolished on 31 March 2009 and its responsibilities in England broadly subsumed by the CQC.

2004. **Quality and Outcomes Framework (QoF).** The reformulated GP contract put an increased emphasis on performance-related pay particularly in relation to the management of chronic disease.

2004. **Clinical.** First Daily Acute Medical (Outpatient) Clinic (AMC) in UK (in Coventry). AMCs later became known as Ambulatory Emergency Clinics (AECs) or Ambulatory Emergency Care Units (AECUs) and are now being renamed as Same Day Emergency Clinics (SDECs).

2004. **Scandal.** Alder Hey, leading to Human Tissue Act 2004. The Alder Hey organ scandal involved the unauthorised removal, retention, and disposal of human tissue, including childrens' organs, between 1988 and 1995. The Act now regulates these activities including prohibiting the sale of human organs.

2004. **Public Health.** Health Protection Agency (HPA) was set up to protect the public in England from infectious diseases and environmental hazards. On 1 April 2013, it was subsumed by Public Health England.

2004. **Monitor** was set up to ensure healthcare provision by Foundation Trusts in England was financially effective. It merged with the Trust Development Agency (TDA) in 2016 to form NHS Improvement.

2005. Three of the four **Standing Advisory Committees** were abolished by the NHS (Standing Advisory Committees) Amendment Order 2005. Why this did not include the dental committee - which was abolished five years later, in 2010 - is unclear.

2005. **Information Technology.** The Health and Social Care Information Centre (HSCIC) was created by merging parts of the NHSIA and the Prescribing Support Unit. It was part of the DH Informatics Directorate, with the role of maintaining and developing the NHS IT infrastructure.

The NHS agency Connecting for Health (CfH) was also formed out of the disassembling of NHSIA. This adopted the responsibility of delivering the NHS National Programme for IT (NPfIT); an initiative to move the NHS in England towards a single, centrally mandated electronic care record connecting GPs to hospitals. In 2013, NHS CfH was disbanded, and some responsibilities taken over by HSCIC.

2005. **NHS Blood and Transplant** was established to take over the responsibilities of UK Transplant (Organ Donation and Transplantation) and the National Blood Service (Blood Donation).

2005. **Mental Health.** The landmark Mental Capacity Act 2005 provided a statutory framework for actions on behalf of adults who lack mental capacity.

2005. **Public Health.** 'Scores on the Doors' Food Hygiene Ratings became part of food hygiene information collected by Local Authorities.

2006. **'Patient Choice'** gave patients the choice of four or five hospitals, ending the tradition of being referred to the local hospital by your GP.

2006. **Reorganisation (Minor).** The 28 sub-regional HAs were reduced to 10 regions. The current arbitrary 7 regions of NHSE are the descendants of the 'original' 1948 fourteen Regional Health Boards, via these 10 regions in 2006 (and other regions at other stages of NHS history).

2006. **Public Health.** Bowel Cancer Screening Programme (BCSP) invited people aged 60-69 years to use a home screening kit.

2006. **Public Health.** NHS Health Act 2006 saw smoking in workplaces and enclosed public spaces made illegal; in Scotland in March 2006, in Wales and Northern Ireland in April 2007, and in England in July 2007. Along with the seat-belt law (1983), this is one of the most important public health measures of all time. The Act also encompassed Forensic Mental Healthcare and created the NHS Counter Fraud Authority.

2007. Public Health. Junk Food Advertising Banned during children's TV programmes. In February 2019, a similar ban across the Transport for London network came into force.

2007. Information Technology. 'NHS Choices' health information website launched. It was integrated with the NHS Direct website and since then - as the NHS website - has been the principle one for NHS health advice in England.

2008. Public Health. Abdominal aortic screening was introduced and offered to men in their 65th year.

2008. Mental Health. The Improving Access to Psychological Therapies (IAPT) Programme was set up to make it easier to access talking therapy on the NHS for people suffering from depression and anxiety disorders.

2008. High-Quality Care for All: the NHS Next Stage (Darzi) Review intended to shift the emphasis of the NHS from increasing the quantity of care to improving its clinical quality. Patients' rights and responsibilities were to be set out in a new NHS Constitution. A workforce strategy was intended to improve the skills and career progression of staff. NHS Evidence, a database within NICE, was also established.

2008. Public Health. The Human Papillomavirus HPV Vaccination for Girls aged 12-13 years was introduced. This has since been offered to boys from 2019.

2009. Pandemic. Swine Flu: this was the second of two pandemics involving H1N1 influenza virus (the first being the 1918-1920 Spanish Flu pandemic). It is estimated to have caused 150,000 to 575,000 deaths globally.

2009. Mixed-sex Hospital Accommodation ended.

2009. NHS Constitution set out the enduring character of the NHS as comprehensive and equitable; and empowered staff and the public to know and exercise their rights to help drive improvements.

The 4 Hour A&E, 18 Week Outpatient Referral and 2 Week Cancer NHS targets were added as rights in March 2010.

2009. Public Health. The Stroke Act F.A.S.T. ('Face, Arm, Speech, Time') campaign was launched.

2009. Public Health. Care Quality Commission (CQC), new regulator for health, mental health and adult social care was formed, evolving out of the Health Commission.

2009. Public Health. NHS Health Checks aim to assess and reduce the risk of heart disease, stroke, type 2 diabetes and kidney disease in individuals between 40 and 74 years who haven't already been diagnosed with a long-term condition.

The 2010s
- MERS-Coronavirus
- Genome project
- 'Lansley' reforms, leading to NHS England and CCGs, and public health returning to local government
- Mental health targets started
- Ebola showed dangers of viruses
- 'Mid-Staffs scandal' showed consequences of over-focus on targets
- 7DS programme and junior doctors' strike
- STPs and tobacco control.

2010. **'Equity and Excellence: Liberating the NHS'** white paper attempted to strengthen provision nationally establishing the NHS Commissioning Board (later NHS England) and the Public Health Service (later Public Health England); and locally establishing Health and Wellbeing Boards. A commitment to 'GP Consortia' and clinically-led commissioning was made. Middle-tier organisations, i.e. Strategic Health Authorities (SHAs) and Primary Care Trusts (PCTs), were abolished.

2011. **Health and Social Care Bill** gave effect to the policies in the 'Equity and Excellence' white paper.

2011 (April-June 2011). **NHS Modernisation: Listening Exercise and NHS Future Forum.** The Bill included safeguards against cherry picking and price competition. GP Consortia become Clinical Commissioning Groups (CCGs), which were required to have governing bodies including at least one nurse and one specialist doctor. From June to September 2011 further scrutiny of the bill paved the way for the HSC Act 2012.

2011. **NHS Reorganisation (Minor).** The 10 SHAs became 4 'SHA Clusters': London, North of England, Midlands (including East of England), and South of England. These became the 4 Regions of NHS England in 2013.

2012. There was an outbreak of **Middle East Respiratory Syndrome Coronavirus (MERS-CoV)** derived from dromedary camels (probably transmitted via bats), in the Middle East; it had a 35% mortality rate and was followed by another outbreak in South Korea in 2015 - further pre-warnings for C19.

2012. The grand Opening Ceremony of the **London 2012 Olympic Games** included a homage to the NHS.

2012. **Public Health.** 100,000 Genomes Project. Plans were announced to introduce DNA mapping for cancer patients and 190 'rare' diseases, including many inherited heart conditions.

2013. **NHS Reorganisation (Major).** The Health and Social Care Act 2012 created NHS England (NHSE) to oversee the budget, planning, delivery and day-to-day operation of commissioning and contracts for GPs and NHS dentists in England.

The Act put more focus on public health and was also designed to strengthen commissioning. It also increased democratic accountability and public voice; with public health responsibilities transferred back to local government.

The C19 Pandemic of 2020 made it (painfully) unclear which agency was (and is) responsible for infectious disease prevention and control. Why? Local public health departments report to (and are part of) the council, and thus above that, the Department for Levelling Up, Housing and Communities (DLUHC). But nationally PHE, is allied to (but not a part of) NHSE and managed by the DHSC (see later).

2013. **Trust Development Agency (TDA)** was formed to monitor the performance and financial management of non-Foundation Trust hospitals, merging in 2016 with Monitor to form NHS Improvement.

2013. **Epidemic.** Western African Ebola Virus Epidemic (2013-2016) caused 11,300 deaths globally, with a mortality of 40%.

2013. **Scandal.** Mid Staffordshire NHS Foundation Trust: The Francis Report found the poor care of patients and high death rates at Mid Staffordshire NHS Foundation Trust from 2010 onwards, were due to an NHS wide over-focus on targets.

2013. **NHS Services, Seven Days a Week Forum** led by Sir Bruce Keogh, Medical Director of NHSE, produced 10 NHS Clinical Standards for a Seven Day Service. This led to a focus on four priority standards in 2015: Time to consultant review, Diagnostics, Consultant directed interventions and Daily consultant-directed review.

2014. In January 2014 the **Duty of Candour** definition, recommended by Francis, was published by the CQC. This sets out the legal duty to be open and honest when things go wrong.

2014. **Health Select Committee's Report on Public Health England** (after its first 7 months) raised concerns PHE staff did not feel able to contradict government policy.

2014. **'Five Year Forward View'**, an NHSE plan, identified the need for a radical upgrade in preventative medicine and public health; supporting national action on obesity, alcohol and other major health risks.

2015. **'Devo Manc'.** Greater Manchester became a pioneer project site for the devolution of NHS functions, intended to enable localities to integrate health and social services.

2015. **Staff Numbers.** NHS became the world's fifth largest employer with 1.7 million staff.

2015. **Mental Health.** Mental Health Targets. By April 2016, 75% of people referred to the IAPT programme in England were to begin treatment within 6 weeks; and greater than 50% of people experiencing a first episode of psychosis, were to start treatment within 2 weeks. This was formalised in an NHSE document 'Achieving Better Access to Mental Health Services by 2020' (October 2014).

Mental Health Target for Eating Disorders. 95% of children and young people referred should receive NICE-approved treatment within 1 week if the case is urgent, and 4 weeks non-urgent.

2015. **Junior doctors' strike.** A junior doctors' contract dispute in England, started in 2012, between NHS Employers and the British Medical Associate (BMA); partly as a response to the 7-day service standards of 2013.

2016. **NHS Improvement (NHSI)** was formed by the merger of Monitor and the TDA, with responsibility to oversee NHS hospitals and independent providers providing NHS-funded care.

2016. **Public Health.** Tobacco Control. The UK Tobacco and Related Products Regulations implemented the European Union Tobacco Products Directive, bringing in larger picture health warnings and other changes.

2017. **Public Health.** PrEP (Pre-exposure Prophylaxis) to Prevent HIV was made available to 10,000 people in England as part of the IMPACT trial. When taken according to instructions, it reduces the risk of HIV transmission to almost zero.

2018. **Public Health.** Fixed-odds Betting Terminals stake limit was reduced to £2.

2018. **Public Health.** Minimum Unit Pricing on alcohol was introduced in Scotland.

2018. **Public Health.** 'Opt-out' Organ Donation.

2019. **NHS Long Term Plan.** This is the current ten-year plan for the NHS in England. The plan aims to deliver improved health in early childhood, provide early diagnosis and prevention of major health problems, increase investment in mental health, and support people to age well. The plan also includes a focus on how to better employ data and digital technology in the NHS.

2019. **Information Technology.** NHSX was created in February 2019 and has oversight of digital strategy and policy in NHS England.

2019. **Information Technology.** NHS App was launched in January, enabling patients to access some of their GP record, organise appointments and renew prescriptions. This became significantly more popular in 2021, when it enabled the public to demonstrate their C19 vaccinations.

2019. **NHS Reorganisation (Minor).** NHS England's Four Regions Split. Four NHSE regions were split into seven.

2019. **NHS Reorganisation (Minor).** NHS England and NHS Improvement to merge.

The 2020s
Decade so far dominated by C19 Pandemic.

2020. **Public Health.** Abortion (Northern Ireland) Regulations 2020. Abortion was decriminalised in Northern Ireland.

2020. **COVID-19 Pandemic.** A new strain of coronavirus, SARS-Cov-2, was first identified in Wuhan, Hubei province, China, in late December 2019. It caused a Severe Acute Respiratory Syndrome, like SAR-Cov and MERS-Cov (other coronaviruses).

On 11 March 2020, the World Health Organisation declared it a pandemic. Globally, over 6 million people have died.

The UK has been devastated with over 143,000 deaths in a population of 67 million, as of November 2021. This is about 40x worse (pmp) than Australia, with approximately 1.450 deaths out of a 27 million population: raising serious questions about the fitness of the health system, particularly in its public health capability.

Despite these failings, the pandemic has led to a groundswell of public support for 'our NHS' including the national 'Clap for our Carers'. 'Protect the NHS' as a key slogan. Homes, shops and parks across the country displayed rainbow symbols to show gratitude to the health service.

Professors Chris Whitty (Chief Medical Officer, CMO), Sir Patrick Valance (Chief Scientific Officer) and Jonathan Van Tam (Deputy CMO), advised by the SAGE (Scientific Advisory Group for Emergencies) panel of experts, became household names.

Three waves of the pandemic had happened by November 2021, the last one being significantly ameliorated by a successful vaccination programme. In the UK at that time, 80% had been 'double vaccinated' at that time.

2020. **Public Health.** Public Health England to be dissolved. In August 2020, it was announced during the C19 pandemic, that PHE was to merge with the NHS Test and Trace service and the Joint Biosecurity Centre to form a new agency, the National Institute for Health Protection (NIHP), under a single leadership team. The new agency would start work immediately to lead England's ongoing response to the pandemic. It was planned to start operating formally from Spring 2021, with a primary focus on public health protection and infectious disease capability.

2021. **Public Health.** UK Health Security Agency (UKHSA) formed. This replaced the NIHP and started work in April 2021. Its first Chief Executive was Dr Jenny Harries.

Further reading

The Nursing Times: paper regarding primary care Groups and Trusts.

https://www.nursingtimes.net/archive/primary-care-groups-and-trusts-08-11-2001/

The King's Fund explain Foundation Trusts.

https://www.kingsfund.org.uk/blog/2016/02/foundation-trust-model

This is the Nuffield Trust's page analysing waiting times in Emergency Departments.

https://www.nuffieldtrust.org.uk/resource/a-e-waiting-times

Chapter 3

Services, Buildings and Funding

"The NHS is a complex system, which can sometimes make it difficult to understand – especially working out who is responsible for what" (NHS England).

This chapter, with Chapter Five (Organisations), tries to explain it.

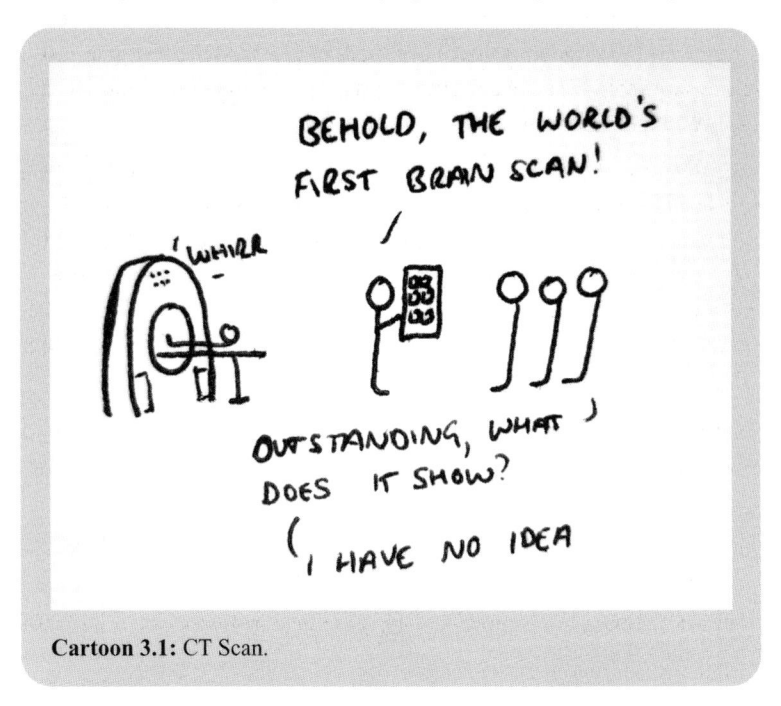

Cartoon 3.1: CT Scan.

Primary, Secondary, Tertiary Care

When the NHS was formed, there were three pillars: GPs (primary care), Hospitals (secondary care) and 'everything else' (run by the council). The hospital pillar is now divided into secondary and tertiary care.

Primary Healthcare

Most patients have contact with this tier first. Preventative healthcare, health promotion, and chronic disease management are its main responsibilities. This care does not require a *specialist* and these services are led by a General Practitioner (GP). Most GPs are independent, self-employed and operate in groups or partnerships. They are not employed directly by the

NHS (with salaries) but deliver services contracted by the NHS. They also benefit from the NHS pension scheme, and grants to improve their premises amongst other things.

There is a tendency for GP partnerships to join up as 'at scale providers' which helps with things like office functions. GP partnerships are currently organised into 'Primary Care Networks' which serve populations of 30-50,000.

Other health professionals - including Practice and District Nurses, IAPT practitioners (Mental Health), Nurse Practitioners, Physician's Associates, Midwives and Health Visitors, Paramedics and Pharmacists, Dentists, Opticians, First Contact Practitioners (physiotherapists) and Podiatrists - also provide primary care services. Like GPs, they are mainly self-employed and only partially funded by the NHS.

Secondary Healthcare

Patients with potentially more serious disease, or advanced symptoms, may be referred by a GP to secondary care, e.g. a hospital clinic, to see a more specialist doctor (or an AHP, e.g. a dietician or physiotherapist). Or, if the patient is very unwell, the GP may decide to admit the patient to hospital via A&E; or get them seen by a hospital specialist that day, e.g. in a medical or surgical admission unit, rapid-access chest pain, fracture or antenatal clinic.

Tertiary Healthcare

When secondary care is unable to provide all the needs of a patient, they can be referred (or transferred) to a regional tertiary healthcare facility (usually a large university-based 'teaching hospital'). A teaching hospital can serve 3-5 'feeder' secondary care hospitals with its services including dialysis/transplantation, cardiac and neurosurgery, cancer treatment and other complicated treatments or procedures. But as most teaching hospitals also provide local secondary care, the distinction between them and secondary care hospitals is blurred.

How these three levels inter-relate is illustrated in Figure 1 above, with the example of diabetes.

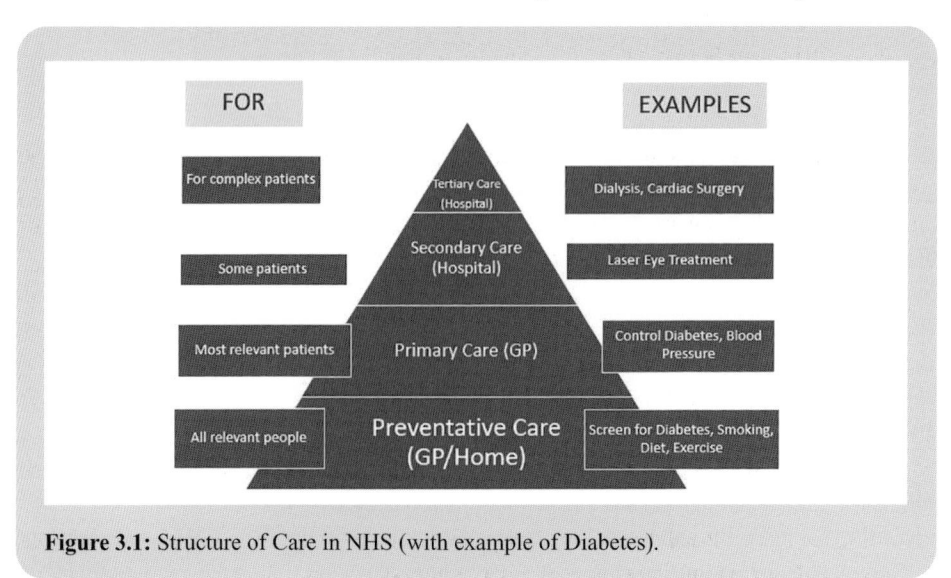

Figure 3.1: Structure of Care in NHS (with example of Diabetes).

Primary Care
General Practice
A general practice is the frontline of the NHS from where GPs can see patients face-to-face in the surgery, at home or, increasingly, virtually. They prescribe drugs, perform minor surgery, and often form an emergency point of call during the working week (and often 'out of hours'). In 2003, the 'new GP Contract' allowed GPs to remove their responsibility for out-of-hours care. District nurses and others may be linked to a practice (and work 'out of' them) without being employed by them.

GPs focus on holistic health combining physical, psychological and social aspects of care. They aim to keep people at home, often working with specialist colleagues (e.g. care of the elderly specialists, psychiatrists and social workers) co-ordinating 'packages of care' for more complex patients. GPs refer around 5% of the patients they see to secondary or tertiary care for assessment and treatment - acting as the *gatekeepers* of the NHS.

Workload

There are over 28,300 FTE (fulltime equivalent) GPs in England, working in over 9,300 practices. Each GP has about 2,100 patients registered to them. General practice provides over 300 million patient consultations each year, compared to 23 million A&E visits. 90% of patient first contacts are with a GP, but GPs receive a little less than 10% of the NHS budget.

GPs, unlike hospitals, are not allowed to discharge registered patients, and would usually not want to (as everyone needs a GP); and their presence on the practice list guarantees income. If they have a difficult, challenging or rude patient, there is little they can do about it.

A typical GP appointment lasts 10 minutes, during which time the GP needs to assess the patient, perhaps including an examination, and initiate a treatment plan. Most GPs provide a service Monday to Friday, from 8am to 6-8pm. A few offer a weekend morning service. Previously many GPs closed on Wednesday or Thursday afternoon[7]. In smaller practices, this was often the GP's only time off in the week[8].

Chronic Disease

General practice plays a significant role in managing chronic disease, e.g. cardiovascular (such as ischaemic heart disease), metabolic (diabetes) and respiratory diseases (COPD) and mental health problems (depression). They may run special clinics for patients with chronic conditions such as asthma, hypertension and diabetes.

Preventative Medicine and Health Promotion

An important part of the work is preventative medicine and health promotion; including child immunisation, smoking cessation and lifestyle advice during consultations. GPs

---

7. It was not always a Wednesday or Thursday. In small market towns, it may have been the day of the market.
8. AS's father was a GP and their home a general practice. Thursday pm was his father's only real 'time off'. Patients sometimes knocked on the front door at weekends.

also have a vital role to play in safeguarding 'at risk' children and adults; and involving appropriate agencies through multi-disciplinary working.

National screening programmes are arranged or coordinated through general practice for pre or early cancerous conditions, e.g. cervical, breast, and bowel screening.

End-of-Life (or palliative care) is often coordinated in primary care in partnership with district nurses, hospices and specialist cancer care nurses, e.g. Macmillan or Marie Curie Nurses.

Regarding C19, many GPs now lead clinical hubs (where patients are seen) and vaccination centres.

Finance in GP

GPs are self-employed and are paid by the number of patients on their list (through a 'General Medical Services (GMS)' contract). Under the GMS contract, there is no incentive to see, investigate or treat patients, encouraging a balanced healthcare provision and efficient use of resources. However, GPs can receive incentive payments for undertaking work outside the GMS contract, e.g. via the Quality and Outcomes Framework (QOF) which encourages preventative medicine, or the 'Universal Offer'.

Most GP buildings are owned by the senior (partner) GPs. Practices also employ 'salaried' GPs, and long or short-term locums. The latter are paid more, to reflect the transient 'on-demand' nature of their work, and lack of job security. There are also 'GPs in training' (called registrars), and medical students, who may work within a practice.

Other staff employed in GP practices include practice managers, nurses, an IT manager (in bigger practices), administration staff and cleaners. Other health professionals may also work there including physician associates who also see patients independently, and paramedics, who may do home visits. GP practices are small businesses that must make money, to pay all their staff. Other ways GPs earn money include onsite pharmacies and doing medical examinations for insurance companies.

Another practice model is an APMS (Alternative Provider Medical Service). This is (usually) based on a fixed term contract issued by a local NHS administration group (Clinical Commissioning Group, CCG) to a third-party provider, to fill gaps in GP provision or target specific population needs.

Summary

GPs see patients from the new-born to the elderly - the 'cradle to grave' ideology. The relationships GPs establish with patients, and the continuity of care provided, is one of the most important aspects of the NHS.

GP Organisations
Primary Care Network (PCN)

PCNs bring together GPs and a range of health and social care professionals - including pharmacy, community, mental health, acute trusts, social care and the voluntary sector - to provide enhanced personalised and preventative care.

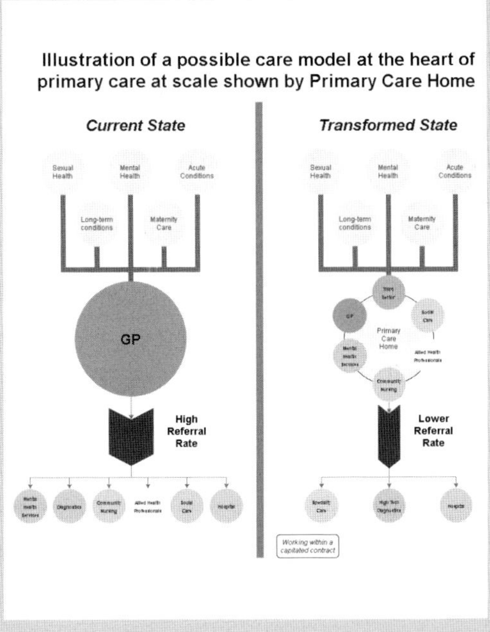

The core characteristics of a PCN are:
- Linked general practices with other local health and care providers, that make geographical sense
- Typically comprise a defined patient population of 30,000-50,000 people (5-10 GP practices)
- Match different needs including flexible access to support for 'healthier' sections of the population, and 'joined up' care for complex conditions
- Focus on prevention and personalised care by connecting statutory and voluntary services
- Better use of data and technology
- Better use of collective resources across practices - potentially increasing hours of access
- In the future, may advise Integrated Care Systems (ICSs, see Chapter 5).

Figure 3.2: Illustration of possible Primary Care Network.

One objective of PCNs is to reduce the referral rate to secondary care, through better use and sharing of resources, as shown in Figure 3.2.

Federation/Association (of GPs)

A GP federation is a less formal grouping of practices which can be single businesses themselves, with their partners having shares. A federation may, for example, coordinate local primary care education, carry out specific health programmes (e.g. vaccination programmes), or provide expertise for health checks (say for populations with learning disabilities) - on behalf of its member practices.

Walk-in Centres

Introduced in 2000, 'walk-in centres' typically allow patients to access care from a GP or nurse without registering or pre-booking. The original idea was that services were to be provided for extended hours (typically 7am to 10pm), 365 days a year; and be sited in accessible locations, such as town centres or adjacent to Emergency Departments (EDs).

Walk-in centres go by many names such as 'NHS walk-in centre', 'walk-in centre', 'GP-Led health centre', 'equitable access centre', 'open access centre', '8 to 8 centre', 'same day centre', 'health centre', 'medical centre', and 'primary care centre'. There are also 'UTCs' and 'UCCs' which are similar and described later. The huge range of services and variable names leads to confusion. So the public often end up going to the ED.

Nurse-led Walk-in Centres

Nurse-led centres may provide some of these services:
- Health advice and information
- Assessment, diagnosis and initial therapy for deep vein thrombosis (DVT) upon referral from GPs
- Blood tests, emergency contraception or travel vaccinations
- Issuing prescriptions
- Minor Injuries, as well as wound care including dressings and the removal of sutures
- X-ray services.

Generally, nurse-led centres provide for a single episode of care, although they may treat patients with symptoms of chronic conditions.

GP-led Walk-in Centres

GP-led centres can offer many of the same services as nurse-led centres. While all walk-in centres provide basic advice and treatment for minor conditions, the full range of services on offer vary greatly by location. Non-registered patients cannot, for example, receive regular treatment for chronic conditions; and are encouraged to see their GP for such care.

Urgent Treatment/Care Centres (UTC/UCC)

An urgent treatment centre is a facility providing urgent medical attention, in non-life-threatening situations. They are often run by GPs and based in or near an ED. Currently, the NHS offers a confusing mix of walk-in centres, UCCs, minor injury units and UTCs. There is some rationalisation of services happening, such that these centres will either be called UTCs, or change to offer other primary healthcare services in a more consistent manner. They will be GP-led and open for at least 12 hours every day. They will be equipped to diagnose and treat many of the common ailments for which people attend EDs.

Minor Injury Units (MIU)

MIUs were often once EDs but now offer limited ED services including simple x-rays.

NHS111 and 'Talk before you walk

Out of hours care is changing rapidly, especially during the C19 pandemic, with many services not now branded as 'urgent care'. So patients may receive an appointment via 111 to get seen in the most appropriate place depending on the problem, e.g.:

- Headache, mild recent general illness - self-care or local pharmacy
- Longstanding symptoms like hip pain or indigestion - GP appointment
- Chest pain, collapse, fit, significant haemorrhage - ED or 999.

Non-practice based GP

New virtual, non-practice based, GP services are being established, especially in larger cities to increase accessibility. One such service is 'Babylon' in which patients can transfer their registration from a conventional GP to a virtual one. In this system, they will initially be assessed via telephone or video by any GP.

This type of GP does not carry out preventative medicine or have links to midwives and health visitors. Though they may offer virtual monitoring of long-term conditions and have clinics where patients can visit to be examined.

They are suitable for adults in middle life with few long-term problems. However, they lack continuity, easy examination capability and follow-up. Babylon charges a patient an annual registration fee or will charge for a one-off assessment.

Pharmacists and Prescriptions

Pharmacies are an important component of primary care with, on average, 1.6 million people visiting a pharmacy in England every day, i.e. double the number visiting GPs. Many feel they are an under-used resource. Pharmacists are highly trained and registered with the General Pharmaceutical Council.

Pharmacists, working in the community, typically supply and dispense medicines but increasingly provide services such as: blood tests (including anticoagulation monitoring and adjustment); vaccinations, and counselling for vaccinations; sexual health advice; smoking cessation advice; and healthy lung screening.

One of the main benefits of community pharmacists is accessibility with at least 11,600 pharmacies in England; many conveniently placed in areas where people live, do their shopping and work.

As part of 'Covid-changes', patients that attend a GP's reception with a minor problem, can now be redirected formally to a 'clinical pharmacy' that is linked to the practice (i.e. information can be exchanged).

Prescription Charges

When the NHS started in 1948, prescriptions were free. As the cost of the NHS spiralled, the power to make a charge was introduced in the NHS Amendment Act 1949; and proposals for charges were a factor in the resignation of Aneurin Bevan from the Labour Government in 1951.

Currently the NHS prescription charge is £9.35 per item. The money raised through the prescription charge is relatively small, equal to 0.5% of the NHS resource budget. In England, in 2013, over 90% of prescription items were dispensed free of charge. About 65% of these were due to age exemption, comprising 60% aged 60 years and over, and 5% children or 16-18 year-olds in full-time education. Prescriptions are also free for people who are pregnant (and 12 months post pregnancy); have specific exempt medical conditions or disabilities (e.g. undergoing cancer treatment); or receive certain state benefits, including a war pension. Contraceptives are also free, as are prescriptions in hospitals.

Prescriptions are free in the three nations of Wales, Scotland and Northern Ireland.

Note: In England, a yearly Prescription Pre-payment Certificate (PPC) costs £108.10 and can save the patient a lot of money.

Dentistry

Dentistry is the treatment of diseases and other conditions affecting the teeth and gums, including the repair and extraction of teeth and the insertion of artificial ones.

General Dental Care

Most dentists work as general dental practitioners (GDPs), usually in a high street practice. Dentistry is unusual in the NHS, as a contribution toward charges by the patient is often required. These charges include emergency treatment as well as three tiers of cost which rise with the complexity of the service provided.

Patients should be able to register with any GDP providing NHS services. However, if assistance is required finding a GDP, your local CCG should be able to help. Similarly 111 may also help find a dentist for urgent symptoms, such as pain outside normal working hours.

Community Dental Care

Dental care is also provided in community settings for patients who have difficulty getting treatment in their high street dental practice. This is because they have specific health related problems, such as severe mental health issues, learning disabilities, dental phobias, or epilepsy, or are elderly or housebound, or require a general anaesthetic. They usually require treatment on a referral basis from a dentist, GP or health professional.

Community dentists work in a variety of locations such as a patient's own home, residential homes, community and mobile clinics - and may be involved in school screening work.

Dental Public Health

Dental public health is a specialty which assesses the dental health needs of a population, and ensures dental services meet those needs. The specialty involves working with people from all branches of dentistry as well as the NHS and other agencies.

Hospital Dental Care

Hospital dental services have five main components:
- Consultant advice and treatment for cases of special difficulty
- Dental care of long-stay hospital in-patients
- Dental care of short-stay patients especially when pain relief is required
- The treatment of certain out-patients (patients on anticoagulants), where it is desirable for the treatment to be carried out in a hospital
- Training dental students and dental nurses.

Hospitals do not provide a dental service to the public, except in the special case of dental hospitals. This is usually free but involves longer waiting and procedure times. Hospital practice is highly specialised and covers:
- Oral and maxillofacial surgery
- Oral surgery
- Orthodontics
- Paediatric dentistry
- Restorative dentistry.

Finance in Dentistry
Dentistry was originally free in the NHS of 1948, but the costs of dental treatment grew rapidly, becoming unsustainable. So, like prescription charges, from 1952, adult patients had to make a financial contribution unless they meet certain exemptions, e.g. pregnancy. The NHS in England spends £3 billion annually (and falling) on primary and secondary care dental services, with over 200,000 patient contacts with NHS dental services per day. The reimbursement to dentists is such that many no longer offer NHS treatment. The dental charge system contributes over £850m (and rising) to the NHS budget last year. This is over twice the income from prescription charges. Dentistry is funded differently in the other three nations of the UK.

The British Dental Association has written a History of Dentistry.

Optometry
Optometrists (known to many as opticians) are the front-line of eye-care in the NHS. This allows them to detect undiagnosed long-term conditions that can cause damage to the eyes such as diabetes or hypertension; during the more than 13 million NHS sight tests across England per year.

Optometrists may work within secondary or primary care. In the community, they perform detailed examinations of the eyes, offering expert advice in relation to eye health and vision. Or they may make a referral for more specialist advice. Optometrists also prescribe glasses and contact lenses and help fit them. Some even provide a hearing aid service.

Optometrists working in hospitals tend to focus on specialist conditions, e.g. glaucoma and macular degeneration. This is as part of multi-disciplinary teams which include specialist eye doctors (ophthalmologists) and specialist nurses.

Finance of Optometry
Like dentistry, eye tests (and some glasses) are partially (and sometimes totally) funded by the NHS, with many adults paying for eye-tests and glasses. Like dentistry and prescriptions, several groups are exempt from charges, including children and people over 60 years, or those with glaucoma. Optometry is funded differently in the other three nations of the UK.

Podiatry
Most podiatry is based in primary care and is not normally funded by the NHS except for certain patients depending on priorities set by the local CCG. It is usually assessed on a

case-by-case basis depending on how serious the condition is, and the individual's risk factors. There are some NHS funded podiatrists working in secondary care. Patients with diabetes, for example, are considered high-risk and have access to NHS podiatry services free of charge.

A podiatrist can provide advice and treatment for conditions such as:
- Painful feet
- Ulcers
- Dry skin; with cracks and cuts on the surface of the skin
- Verrucae and warts
- Scaling and peeling of the soles on feet
- Abnormal gait or deformity.

Citizens Advice provide excellent information on what services can be obtained on the NHS, including podiatry.

STD (Sexually Transmitted Disease) and Rape Crisis Centres
Sexual Health Clinics

Sexual health clinics are also called genitourinary medicine (GUM) or sexual and reproductive health (SRH) services. They usually operate separately outside both GP and acute hospitals because they are often funded, and report to another organisation called a 'Community Trust'. As a result, their clinical information is usually 'hidden' from GPs and hospitals, as well as for privacy reasons. This can be frustrating for the patients and other parts of the NHS, and cause mistakes in their care. For example, GPs and secondary care doctors may be unaware their patient has HIV.

Sexual health clinics offer a wide range of services, including:
- Testing, reassurance and treatment for sexually transmitted infections (STIs)
- Advice and information about sexual health
- Urinary and reproductive health
- Free condoms
- Contraception – including emergency contraception, such as the emergency contraceptive pill, and long-acting contraception, e.g. implants and coils
- Pregnancy testing
- HIV testing and management and counselling
- PEP (post-exposure prophylaxis) – medication that can help prevent people from developing HIV if they have been exposed to it
- Hepatitis B vaccination
- Advice about abortion and unwanted pregnancy
- Help for people who have been sexually assaulted
- If necessary, a referral to another specialist.

Sexual health clinics are open to everyone, either on a drop-in or appointment basis, regardless of age; and may have sessions for specific groups, such as young people, and members of LGBTQ+ community. All services offered are free.

Rape Crisis Centres

Rape Crisis Centres provide specialist support services to people who have experienced rape, sexual violence, or sexual abuse. Some are partially funded by the NHS through CCGs, but also receive funding from local police bodies and authorities. Many centres also provide specialist advocacy services via Independent Sexual Violence Advisors or Advocates (ISVAs).

ISVAs' main role is to provide practical information and emotional support to victims and survivors who have, or are considering, reporting an assault to the police and through and after any court hearings. Cases do not have to be reported to the police for a rape crisis service to be accessed. A crisis advocate also helps with practical issues that might arise from the sexual violence experiences, e.g. they can provide support accessing services like housing, education or health. Like all rape crisis workers, an ISVA will listen and believe the client, and will not put pressure on them to make any decisions (or take any action they are not comfortable with).

Other Examples of Primary Care
Mental Health
The mental health primary care system is described in Chapter 7.

Non-NHS Therapies
The NHS, i.e. the taxpayer, cannot pay for everything, e.g. osteopathy, non-NHS physiotherapy, counselling and acupuncture are outside the NHS.

Secondary and Tertiary Care
Hospitals
'Hospital' is a Middle English word derived from Old French, via the medieval Latin word *hospitale*, from the Latin *hospitalis* (meaning 'hospitable'), from Latin *hospes* ('host, guest, stranger'). They provide a variety of medical and nursing services for people and serve as a centre for investigations and teaching.

Secondary Care

Secondary care is usually provided by smaller local hospitals (often with 300-500 beds), previously called 'District General Hospitals' (DGHs). They have beds for patients with acute (rapid onset and usually short in duration) illnesses (e.g. heart attacks, appendicitis or fractures), maternity services, intensive care and long-term care. Patients are usually referred by primary care health professionals, mostly GPs. Some come from dentists, optometrists and other professionals; or patients may 'self-refer', e.g. to the ED.

Local hospitals have a range of departments, e.g. medical and surgical, and specialist units such as cardiology, neonatal care units and outpatient facilities. They are supported by a pharmacy, pathology laboratories and a radiology department. In recent years, many local hospitals have joined with medical schools and are actively involved in research and teaching.

Treatment for many acute conditions is now provided on a geographical 'network' basis, i.e. smaller local (secondary care) hospitals work with regional teaching (tertiary care) hospitals. So specialist care (with better outcomes) is provided for everyone, not just locals. This is because a journey by ambulance of up to an hour is well tolerated, and the benefits of specialised 'hi-tech' care hugely outweigh the risks of transfer in many conditions, e.g. major trauma, heart attack, and stroke.

Tertiary Care

A 'teaching hospital' is classically a larger regional centre of tertiary care, often with over 800 beds. They are usually in a major city and are affiliated to a medical school. They provide secondary care service to their local population but also offer more specialised services to a wider area. Some of their patients are referred by nearby secondary care hospitals, for specialised care or a treatment they do not provide (e.g. neurosurgery).

They have large specialist academic departments and are known for excellence in research. Teaching hospitals work in larger teams, partly in the community, managing a wider range of patients with complex or rarer conditions compared to local hospitals. Additional services include dialysis and transplantation; cancer treatment (chemotherapy and radiotherapy); vascular, cardiac and neurosurgery; and facilities for major trauma.

Some tertiary care hospitals are even more specialised, including:
- Trauma centres
- Rehabilitation hospitals
- Children's hospitals
- Hyper-specialist hospitals. These include hospitals that focus on a single organ or group of diseases, e.g. Moorfields Eye Hospital (London) and The Christie NHS Foundation Trust (a cancer hospital in Manchester). Sometimes these hyper-specialist hospitals are said to provide Quaternary Care, i.e. they provide a service to Tertiary Care centres that need help with complex patients
- Psychiatric Hospitals - also known as mental health hospitals - and mental health units, specialise in the treatment of serious mental disorders, e.g. major depressive disorder, schizophrenia and bipolar disorder. Psychiatric hospitals vary widely in their size. Mental Health Secondary Care is described in detail in Chapter 7.

Most hospitals in the UK are run by the NHS, with most of their funding coming from the local CCG (see below). The larger teaching hospitals also receive significant funding from the Specialist Commissioning system (see later and Chapter 6). This may account for 30% of their income.

Some other hospitals are run by other health organisations (for profit or non-profit), health insurance companies, or charities - in accordance with the original meaning of the word, hospitals as 'places of hospitality'. And this meaning is preserved in the names of some institutions such as the Royal Hospital Chelsea, established in 1681 as a retirement and nursing home for veteran soldiers.

Typical Hospital Structure
Most hospitals have a four-tier structure, reporting to an executive team:
1. **Board.** Chairperson, and Non-Executive Directors, and some Executives
2. **Senior Management Team.** This includes Executives and other senior staff
3. **Divisions** (examples). Medicine, Surgery, Women's and Children's, Urgent Care and Support. There are groups of similar departments within 5-7 Divisions (or Directorates)
4. **Department** (examples). Cardiology and Respiratory (Medicine); General Surgery, Trauma and Orthopaedics (Surgery); Obstetrics and Gynaecology and Paediatrics (Women's and Children's); Emergency Department and ICU (Urgent Care); Outpatients, Infection Control, Pharmacy, Radiology and Pathology (Support). There are usually 15-25 departments.

There are other (non-clinical) services that work across the hospital in all departments, e.g. information technology, estates, catering, portering, etc. (these may be NHS or private sector). Teaching hospitals may have extra departments like Research and Innovation.

Finance in Hospitals
Hospital finance is complicated. Hospitals are 'providers' of care which is bought by commissioners, or 'purchasers', like CCGs and NHS England. They were paid for the actions they did, e.g. an outpatient appointment or an emergency hospital admission, or an operation or a procedure. This system, the so-called 'purchaser/provider split', was brought in by the Conservative government (endorsed by Labour) more than 30 years ago. The theory that money should 'follow' the patient, is based on what is called 'Payment by Results (or PbR)'[9].

In other words, hospitals were not paid according to their number of staff, or the patients on their 'list'. Rather, PbR created a perverse incentive to do more work, generating a tendency to set up new services (or take over other geographical areas) - and sometimes to over-investigate and treat. This system meant if patients were seen and treated, the CCG or NHS England had to pay for their care. This allowed hospitals to grow and take an increasing proportion of the NHS budget away from other important services, like primary care. Another flaw in this system, unlike a true market, is that the commissioners have a fixed budget from the government. This led to rationing of care, inequity, and budget deficits.

This is why, in recent years, there has been a tendency to go back to an old system called a 'block contract'. In this, a hospital is paid a set amount (say £500 million a year) by a CCG - no matter how much work they do. The disadvantage of this is that it is hard for the purchaser to influence the quality of care.

There is now a move towards Integrated Care Systems (ICSs) where a geographic area receives a pot of money for all care (primary, secondary, some tertiary and social care) and care providers are encouraged (or forced) to collaborate. This may, in time, result in better quality care.

---

9. It was never really payment by *results* (i.e. clinical performance); more payment by activity (what you do).

Private Finance Initiatives
The Private Finance Initiative (PFI) was (and is) a controversial UK government procurement policy aimed at creating 'public-private partnerships'. In such a partnership, private firms are contracted to complete and manage large public projects – such as NHS hospitals – using private money to pay for the upfront costs of their design, build and maintenance. The costs of this borrowing are repaid over many years (like a mortgage), giving the private sector a profit and the NHS a new hospital. The hospital, after 25 years, is then owned by the state.

Other Parts of NHS
Administration
The NHS is subject to constant reorganisation in attempts to satisfy - and reign in - ever-expanding demands consequent upon technological advances, public expectations and an ageing population. The NHS provides a service to society, and every government has the right (and duty) to review how this is provided and funded.

Schools
The role of the school health team is to support healthcare in children, young people and their families/carers in school. The team often consists of healthcare support workers, health visitors, children's nurses, registered nurses, doctors, psychologists and other allied health professionals, e.g. physiotherapists and occupational therapists. Health facilities in schools are inspected against the national standards of the Independent Schools Inspectorate in England.

School Nurses
School nurses are registered nurses who gain additional qualifications to become specialist community public health nurses. They use their additional training to encourage and enable children to make healthy lifestyle choices and to reach their full potential. School nurses, employed directly by a school, should lead and influence the health agenda for the school.

Prisons, Military, etc
The NHS is responsible for providing appropriate healthcare for the complex needs of people detained in settings such as prisons, young offenders' units and immigration centres. People in detention should receive the same level of care and service offered to the rest of the population. The NHS provides primary care, secondary care and public health-related care, such as substance misuse services, in detention settings - as well as dental, ophthalmic and mental health services.

People in detention are more likely to experience health inequalities compared to those in the community. The NHS aims to address some of these inequalities by, for example:
- Encouraging adults to stop smoking and creating a national 'Smoke Free Prison' programme
- Enhance recovery from substance abuse
- Ensuring the adequate delivery of public health screening (bowel screening, prostate screening, Abdominal Aortic Aneurysm screening) and vaccination programmes.

Services, Buildings and Funding

National Institute for Health and Care Excellence (NICE), Care Quality Commission (CQC), Health Education England (HEE) and Public Health England (PHE)

These organisations are not strictly part of the NHS but closely allied to it. Their roles are described further in Chapter 5.

Buildings and Services Closely Linked to NHS
Universities

Universities work closely with the NHS in England through HEE. Before the NHS, health education was seen as something which took place before one began work as a practitioner. The scale of the NHS meant integrating education into the professional setting became easier allowing for 'life-long learning'. A key step towards this was the introduction of a one-year period of 'provisional registration' for newly qualified doctors (house officers), as part of the Medical Act 1950.

Since 1950, on completing medical school, doctors undertook a supervised resident appointment (usually in two 6-month blocks). This is now two years, usually with six 4-month blocks, and the doctors are known as Foundation 1 or 2 ('F1-2s'), or Foundation Year 1 or 2 ('FY1-2s'). The doctor is registered with the GMC after the first year if their performance has been satisfactory, and may legally leave the NHS and work independently, although this is unusual. The training of doctors in the UK is summarised in Figure 3 below.

As well as providing doctors, nurses and pharmacists, and other health professions, universities work with the NHS to develop new skills and ideas. This is often the role of clinical academics, who work at both an NHS hospital and its affiliated university. Their research produces new treatments and methodologies, constantly improving the care on offer.

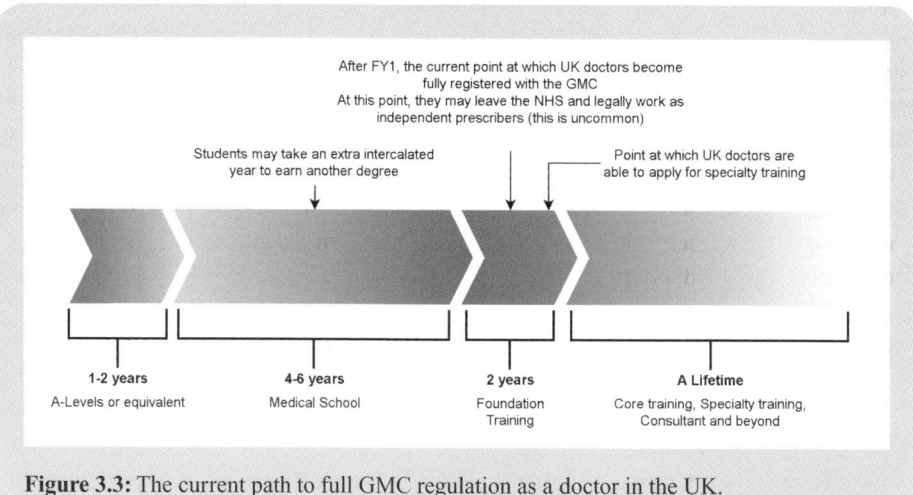

Figure 3.3: The current path to full GMC regulation as a doctor in the UK.

Royal Colleges and Professional Bodies

Most of the medical, nursing, AHP and other professional bodies have base buildings, often in London. Many branches of medicine have Royal Colleges (also in London), some of which are very ancient. They are discussed more in Chapter 5. They have an important inspection role, as well as setting professional exams and standards. For example, if a unit within a hospital, or a general practice, is having problems (especially with performance or staff behaviour), senior management can request a 'College Visit', to get to the bottom of problems, and suggest ways of improving things. They have the power to remove junior or middle grade doctors, if they do not think they are getting adequate supervision or training. Some branches of medicine have professional bodies that are not Royal Colleges.

Local Authority

The local council is responsible for some aspects of healthcare, just as it was in 1948. This currently includes the local public health department. Local authorities have buildings that include these departments. They are responsible for social care, and other services like substance abuse.

Funding and Performance of NHS

Sources

The NHS is funded via general taxation, National Insurance and user charges. General taxation accounts for most of the funding (81%) whilst National Insurance provides 17.9%, and patient charges (prescription and dental) 1.2%. The amount of funds allocated to the NHS each year is determined by central government.

The government distributes these funds to the DHSC (for England) and the NHS in Scotland, Wales and Northern Ireland. In 2018/19 health services expenditure per head was highest in Northern Ireland per year (£2,436) and lowest in England (£2,269). Funds are distributed to the devolved nations according to the *Barnett Formula*.

Most would consider these prices as good value for money, especially when compared to the USA, where the average cost of private health insurance, which most people have, is about £4,000 a year. In the UK, it is estimated about 10% of the population is covered by private medical insurance, but most use the NHS as their primary provider.

Cost

The services described above are not cheap, and the NHS is *not free*. Total UK central government funding in 2018/19 (including spending by central government departments and devolved administrations) was £152.9 billion. Of this total, in 2018/2019, the DHSC spent about 7% of total GDP (Gross Domestic Product), i.e. about 7% of your taxes. If we add the funding for the three nations, this rises to about 9% of GDP. This is in line with other developed countries.

NHSE received the largest amount (£113 billion), as it has the biggest population. £84.5 billion of this budget was allocated to CCGs according to a population and needs-

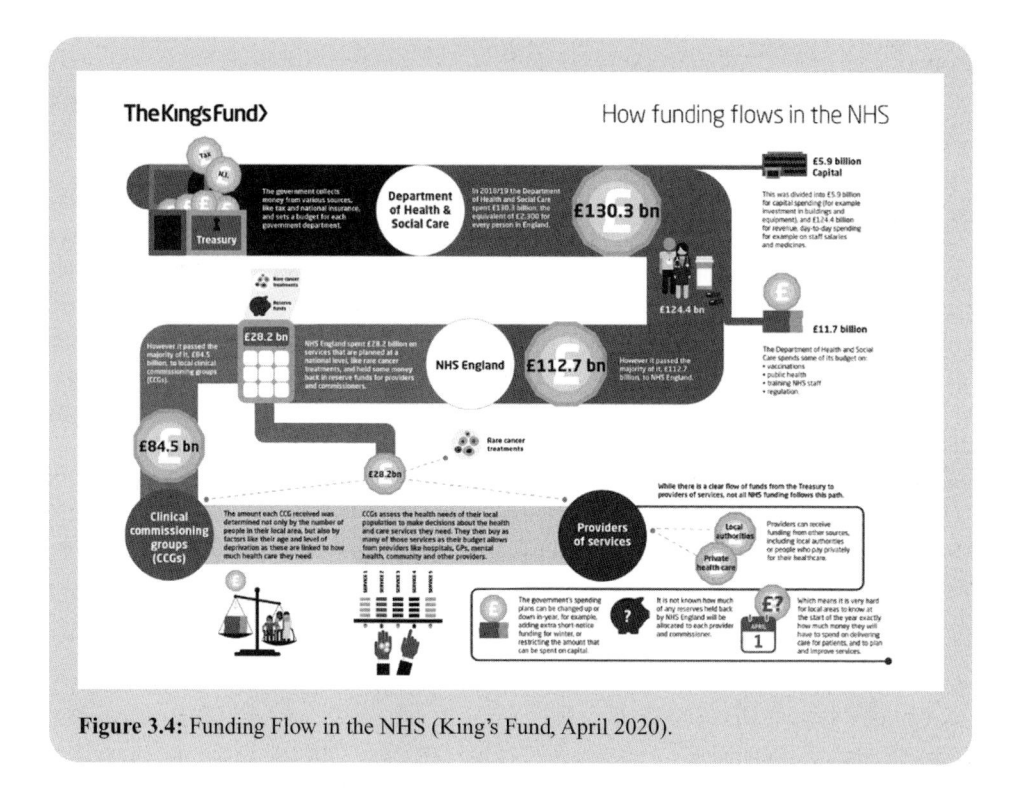

Figure 3.4: Funding Flow in the NHS (King's Fund, April 2020).

based formula. Of the DHSC's 'arms lengths bodies', the largest in terms of investment, are PHE and HEE (receiving £4.0 and £4.4 billion respectively).

NHSE retains around a quarter of the budget for other responsibilities including about £20 billion (16% of the budget) in 2018/19, for Specialised Commissioning (see Chapter 6). The rest funds other services (e.g. PHE, HEE, NICE, CQC, prisons and armed services), and itself.

Pre-C19 pandemic, this meant Specialised Commissioning was one of the fastest growing elements of the NHS budget – increasing by an average of over 7% per year. This is a concern as it means in the future, there will be less funds for 'ordinary' healthcare like GPs, local hospitals and mental health.

How the 2018/19 budget flowed through the system is summarised in the following King's Fund diagram (Figure 3.4).

Cost of Individual Activity
The following list describes the approximate costs of individual contacts with the NHS. The data is from NHS Improvement and shows 2017/18 data.

Day case procedure	£750
Hospital admission (per day)	£350
Ambulance (which takes patient to hospital)	£250

ED attendance	£160
Hospital outpatient appointment	£125
GP attendance	£30

Rising Cost of Healthcare

Since its creation, the annual budget of the NHS has increased steadily in a bid to meet the rising needs and demands of a fast-growing population. Deciding upon the first NHS budget in 1948 was no easy task. The Beveridge Report, the blueprint for the welfare state in 1942, suggested it would cost £130 million. But as the appointed day neared, estimates varied; from £108m in a 1944 White Paper, to £122m in various cabinet papers, and £134m in the NHS bills laid before Parliament. In fact, price rises, higher standards, and simple errors in forecasting demand and costs, meant the actual spend turned out to be £373m. In other words, the NHS now costs over 330 times more than it did in 1948.

From the start it was realised the NHS was not going to be cheap and the public were informed of this in a 1948 leaflet (Figure 3.5), which was sent out to all people in the UK. It said:

"Everyone - rich or poor, man, woman or child - can use it or any part of it. There are no charges, except for a few items. There are no insurance qualifications. But it is not a 'charity'. You are all paying for it, mainly as taxpayers, and it will relieve your money worries in time of illness".

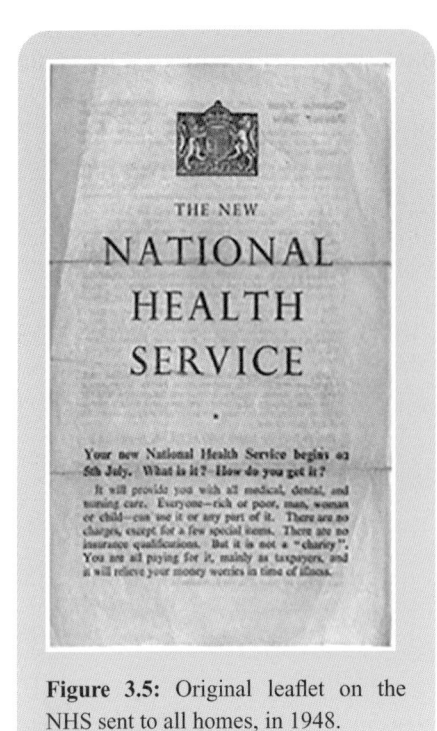

Figure 3.5: Original leaflet on the NHS sent to all homes, in 1948.

This following graph (Figure 3.6) shows the cost of the NHS over the last 60 years, and the % of GDP (Gross Domestic Product), i.e. taxes.

This graph could look quite different in 5 years, when the full impact of C19 will be calculated. Even before C19, the total NHS budget had been increasing rapidly. For NHSE, it would have been £127 billion (pre-C19) in the current financial year (2020-21), £133bn in 2021/22, £140bn in 2022/23 and £148bn in 2023/24. The government is now predicting a DHSC budget of £201.7 billion in 2020/21 (including capital spending).

The NHS in Scotland, Wales and Northern Ireland is being budgeted in 2021/22; for £13.2 billion, £8.0bn and £4.5bn respectively (total £25.7 billion). And large increases are also planned for them, as for England. These figures do not include a C19 prediction.

Services, Buildings and Funding

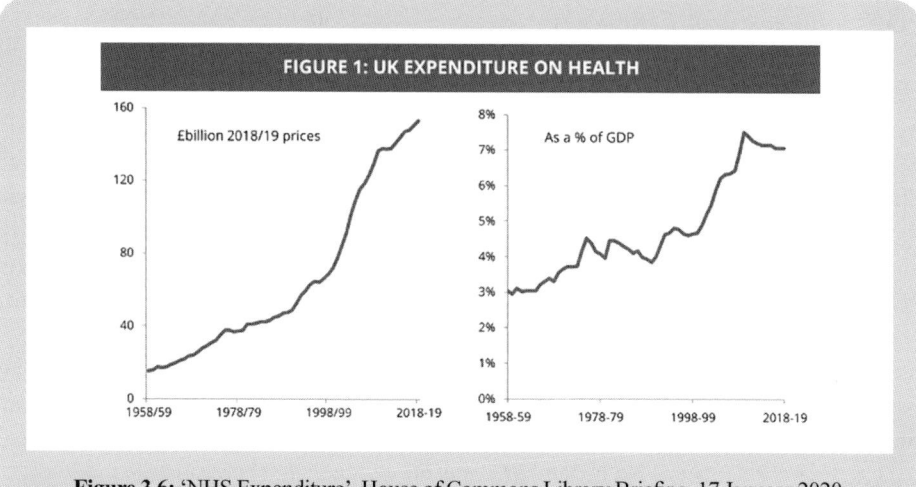

Figure 3.6: 'NHS Expenditure'. House of Commons Library Briefing. 17 January 2020.

Comparison of Health vs Other Government Spending

Health funding, as a proportion of total government spending, is not a huge issue in the UK, as shown in Figure 3.7 below. This because its funding is based on population growth, and the public (and all governments) support and prioritise the NHS.

Despite that, most of the public (and most NHS staff) want more money, as they do for school education. This is understandable. But the advantage of being linked to population growth is considerable. This is because, GPs are paid by the numbers of patients registered, and hospitals by their activity (i.e. what they do). Modern society is complex, and we also need government funding in other areas (justice, defence, transport, social care). So it is constantly necessary to compare NHS funding to what we spend in other areas of society.

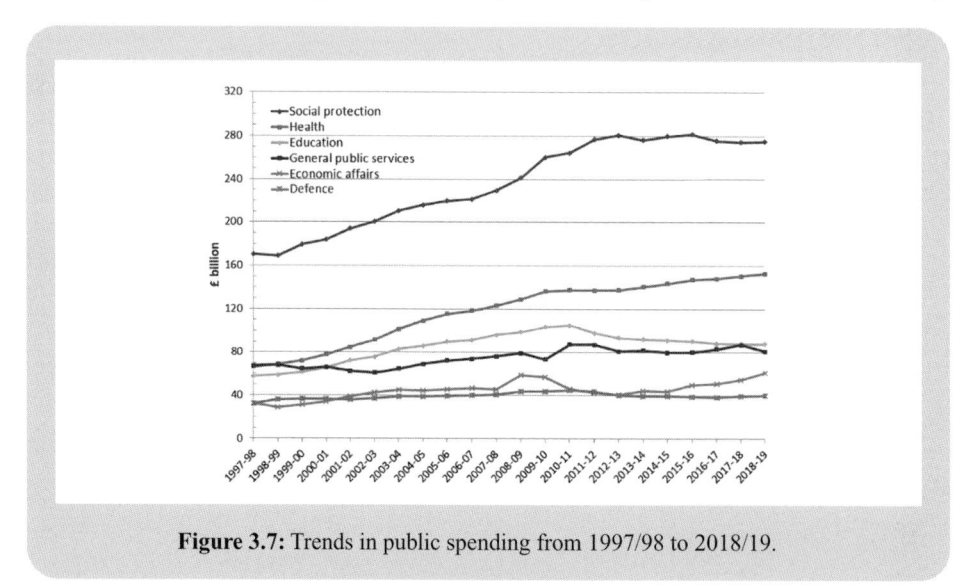

Figure 3.7: Trends in public spending from 1997/98 to 2018/19.

NHS Efficacy and Efficiency

Is the NHS any good? That is a simple but difficult and complex question. We might claim some benefits, e.g. life expectancy at birth has increased between 1948 and 2019; by 13.6 years for men and 12.8 years for women (reaching an average of 79.9 years and 83.6 years, respectively). Additionally, infant and perinatal mortality rates have decreased dramatically (from 34 deaths per 1,000 live births in 1948 to 3.8 deaths per 1,000 live births in 2019). Mortality rates have also reduced for major diseases including respiratory and cardiac diseases and cancer. Whether these improvements are due to the NHS is another issue. Social, societal and economic improvement has happened at the same time, and doubtless, these play a big role in these improvements.

A second question that is almost as hard is, is the NHS efficient? Most agree it is not inefficient and is reasonable value for money. Certainly, the average length of hospital stay for all causes in the UK is 'OK'. It was 6.9 days in 2014. This compares to 16.9 in Japan, 9 in Germany, 7.8 in Italy, 7.6 in New Zealand, 6.6 in Spain and 5.6 in France.

Patient Satisfaction with NHS

Despite its challenges, strengths, weaknesses and cost, a small majority of the public say they are satisfied with the NHS. The British Social Attitudes survey of nearly 3,000 people found 53% of people in England, Scotland and Wales were satisfied with it in 2018

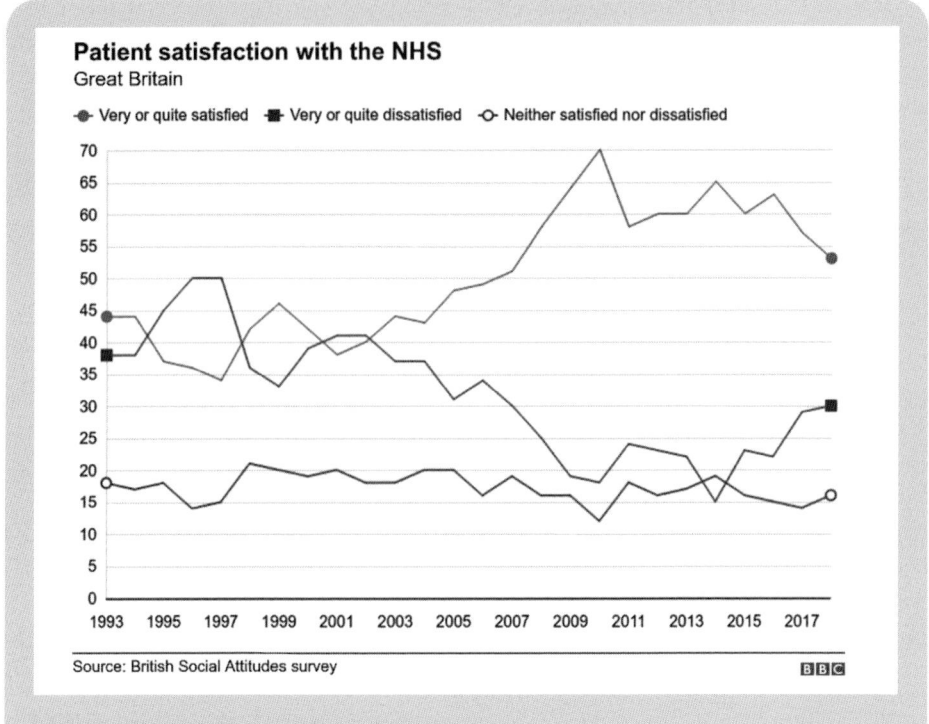

Figure 3.8: British Social Attitudes Survey, 2018.

(see Figure 8 below), but there is a trend towards being less satisfied in the last 10 years. Waiting times and a lack of staff are current major concerns.

Further reading

An NHS guide to the healthcare system in England.

https://assets.publishing.service.gov.uk/government/uploads/system/uploads/attachment_data/file/194002/9421-2900878-TSO-NHS_Guide_to_Healthcare_WEB.PDF

The King's Fund guide to Primary Care Networks.

https://www.kingsfund.org.uk/publications/primary-care-networks-explained

The Nuffield Trust's briefing paper on the structure of the NHS in England.

https://www.nuffieldtrust.org.uk/files/2019-12/parliament-nhs-structure.pdf

Chapter 4

Staff and Training

"It [the NHS] will last as long as there are folk left with the faith to fight for it."
Aneurin Bevan realised the NHS is you, and the importance of its staff.

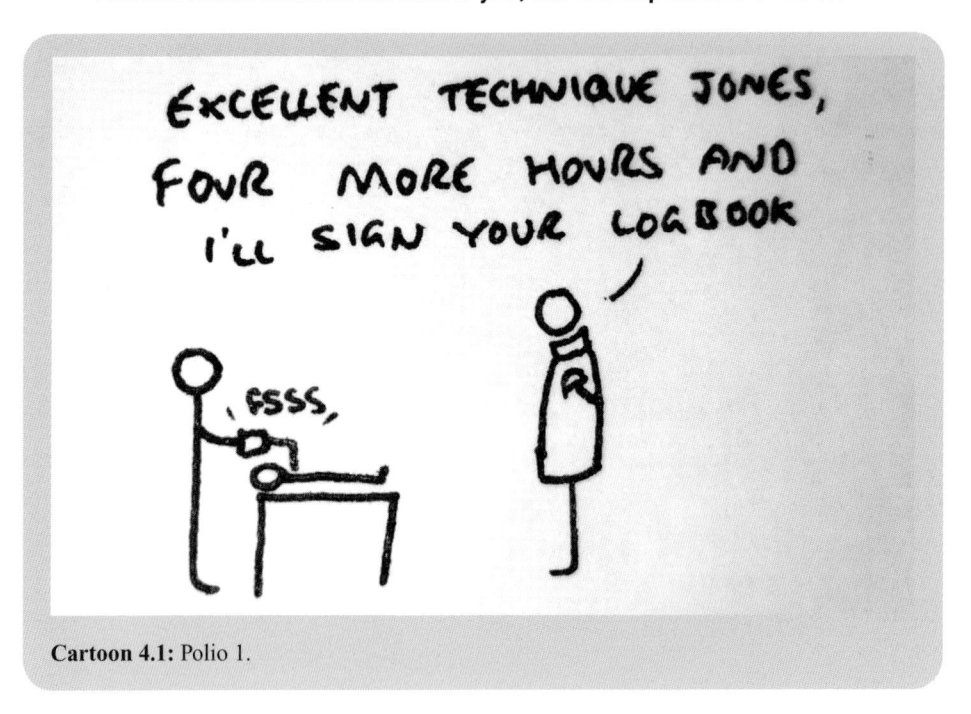

> EXCELLENT TECHNIQUE JONES, FOUR MORE HOURS AND I'LL SIGN YOUR LOGBOOK
>
> FSSS

Cartoon 4.1: Polio 1.

Background

The NHS is thought to be the biggest employer in Europe, and the 5th biggest in the world. It is the second largest single-payer publicly funded healthcare system in the world after the Brazilian 'Sistema Unico de Saude'. In 2020, there were an estimated 1.6 million people working within the NHS. 53.1% of NHSE's workforce are professionally qualified, making it the largest employer of highly skilled professionals in the world.

How big it is, is surprisingly difficult to state, i.e. we don't know the number of fulltime healthcare workers in the NHS, or the number of hospitals or beds, let alone patients. The data above and below are estimates. The number of staff registered are not necessarily all working (and not necessarily in the UK) and may not be full-time. The data also does not include those who work indirectly for the NHS, e.g. estates, catering and staff in PFI hospitals.

We know more about its activity. Every day over 820,000 people (i.e. about 1 in 80 of the population) visit their GP practice or practice nurse, and over 70,000 people (about 1 in 950) visit the ED, of which 13,400 are admitted. To look after these huge numbers, large numbers of staff in many different roles are required. It is not possible to include all of them within this chapter, however the more common roles will be described. More information about careers within the NHS can be accessed on the NHS health careers website.

Why Work in the NHS?
There are four good reasons:

Interest and Fun. Most of us in the NHS enjoy going to work. It is a privilege and an altruistic place to work. Furthermore, it benefits your family and friends. Why? As an employee you understand how the system works. If you care about people and want to be part of a team, the NHS is the great place to work.

Kudos. In surveys, alongside teachers, doctors, nurses and other health professionals, are considered the most respected professions.

Working Conditions. Even though you work hard, and often unsocial hours in the early years, the NHS has reasonable pay and working conditions. These include a generous pension, annual and study leave allowance. It has good terms and conditions if staff become unwell or want to start a family. It is also easy for people later in their career, or having had a family, to work part-time.

Training. Career development is encouraged, with ample opportunity to learn new skills and take new qualifications - which can lead to promotion. In fact, AS knows of a porter who became a Chief Executive!

NHS Agenda for Change
Pay is important. The Agenda for Change (AfC) is the payment system used to standardise most salaries within the NHS. AfC applies to all staff directly employed by the NHS, except for those covered by the Doctors' and Dentists' review body, and very senior managers.

AfC uses a banding system, where staff members are allocated a pay band. The band with the lowest salary is 1 and salaries increase progressively to 8 and 9. Salaries within a band may increase annually for each year of service. The pay rates for each band are regularly updated.

The pay rates for each band are increased in areas where there are high living costs, these are called High-Cost Area Supplements.

Understanding the NHS

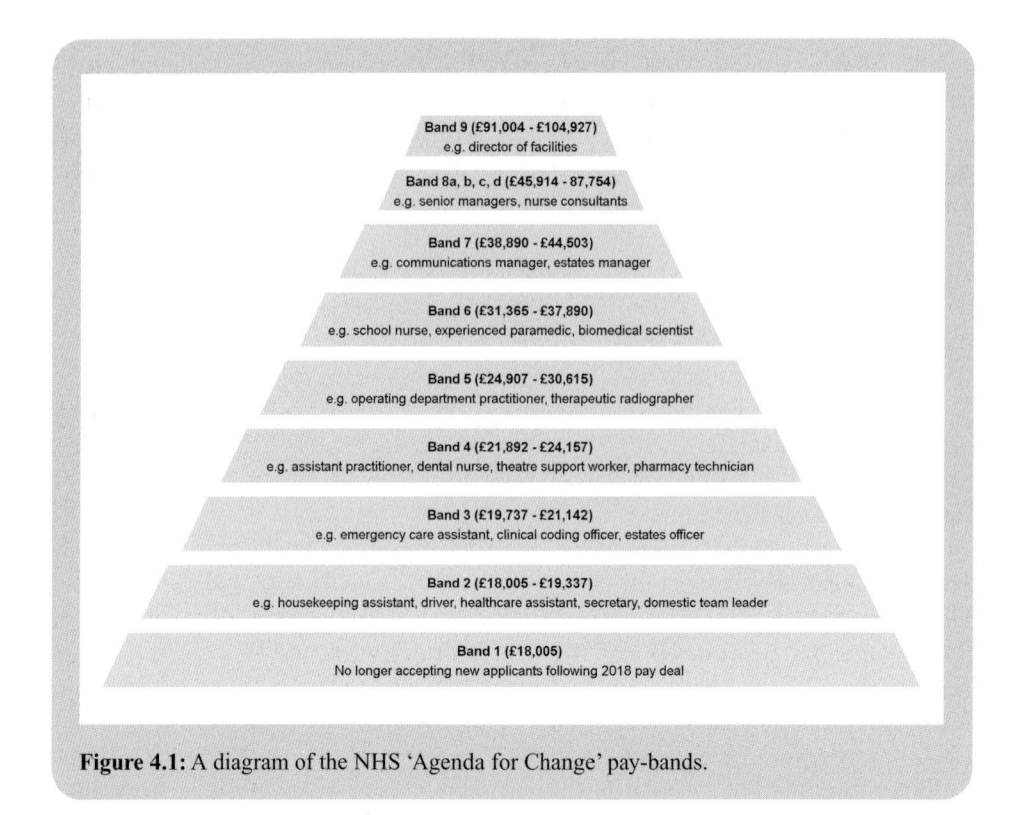

```
              Band 9 (£91,004 - £104,927)
                 e.g. director of facilities
            Band 8a, b, c, d (£45,914 - 87,754)
            e.g. senior managers, nurse consultants
              Band 7 (£38,890 - £44,503)
         e.g. communications manager, estates manager
              Band 6 (£31,365 - £37,890)
    e.g. school nurse, experienced paramedic, biomedical scientist
              Band 5 (£24,907 - £30,615)
     e.g. operating department practitioner, therapeutic radiographer
              Band 4 (£21,892 - £24,157)
 e.g. assistant practitioner, dental nurse, theatre support worker, pharmacy technician
              Band 3 (£19,737 - £21,142)
    e.g. emergency care assistant, clinical coding officer, estates officer
              Band 2 (£18,005 - £19,337)
 e.g. housekeeping assistant, driver, healthcare assistant, secretary, domestic team leader
                   Band 1 (£18,005)
       No longer accepting new applicants following 2018 pay deal
```

Figure 4.1: A diagram of the NHS 'Agenda for Change' pay-bands.

Nurse

Nurses are the largest group of health professionals. As of August 2020 there were over 296,000 employed within the NHS. Figure 4.1 shows the AfC Band Allocation for Nurses' pay (and other NHS Health Professionals).

Adult Nurse

Adult nurses provide care for patients 18 years old and over. An adult nurse looks after a range of patients with differing health conditions, e.g. in a hospital, the community, or GP surgery. Nurses work as part of the multidisciplinary team providing 'hands-on' care.

Day-to-day activities include:
- Administering medication
- Writing and implementing care plans
- Cleaning and dressing wounds
- Procedures, such as, performing ECGs, inserting NG tubes and catheters
- Assisting with patient personal care needs.

Depending on where an adult nurse works, they can do further training (e.g. to undertake other procedures). They can move up to leadership roles including Ward Sister, Modern Matron, up to Chief Nursing Officer.

Nurses who wish to undertake extra academic training can study for a master's level qualification to become Advanced Nurse Practitioners (ANPs). ANPs can independently run clinics, make diagnoses, and prescribe medication. There are ANPs in almost all branches of medicine. ANPs and Advanced Clinical Practitioners (see later) are widely used in Acute Medicine and the ED.

Training
Nurses train for three years to obtain a nursing degree, after which they are registered with the Nursing and Midwifery Council (NMC) and become Registered Nurses (RNs). Those with previous health related degrees can undertake a shortened course or master's level qualification. During this time, nurses will attend lectures and placements, working alongside nurses wherever nursing care is practiced. Many nurses find it useful to have work experience as a Healthcare Assistant (see below) before their training. Some NHS trusts offer nursing degree apprenticeships.

Nursing Associate
Nursing Associates (NAs) are a new role within the NHS. They address the gap between healthcare assistants (see below) and RNs (above) in providing care. NAs can work in any field of care.

Day-to-day activities include:
- Providing support to RNs
- Taking 'observations', e.g. temperature, blood pressure, pulse and respiratory rate
- Sharing information regarding patient's condition with an RN
- Assisting with personal care.

Training
The training to become an NA is a level five 'foundation degree' and is Nursing and Midwifery Council approved. This is often an apprenticeship lasting two years, with one day a week reserved for academic study with the rest on work placement. Since 2018, NAs must also register with the NMC upon completion of their training. They are similar to a previous role called State Enrolled Nurse (SEN).

Healthcare Assistant
Healthcare assistants (HCAs) work within a variety of settings and provide personal care and make sure patients are comfortable. HCAs work under the guidance of healthcare professionals such as nurses or doctors, and depending on where an HCA works, their responsibilities differ but might include:
- Assisting with personal care toileting
- Providing support
- Feeding patients and helping at mealtimes
- Running outpatient clinics, and taking blood.

Training
There are no formal qualifications needed to be an HCA. Some employers may want GCSEs or functional skills level 2 in English & Maths. Many HCAs undertake National Vocational Qualifications or Qualification and Credit Framework courses to develop and progress. There are apprenticeship training roles for HCA too.

Midwife
A midwife is the main healthcare worker responsible for women during pregnancy, birth and in the early postnatal period. Midwives are also able to specialise in certain areas, e.g. mental health.

Midwives can work both in the community and in hospitals. Whilst working in a hospital, midwives may work in the delivery suite, postnatal ward, maternity triage and assessment, or neonatal units. Midwives working in the community may work in various settings, such as in GP practices, children's centres, clinics and within the expectant mothers' homes. Midwives may also support women during labour in their own homes.

Day-to-day working includes:
- Educating and supporting women
- Monitoring foetal development
- Monitoring labour and delivering babies.

Training
Midwives are trained on university courses which are 2-3 years long. The exception is those who are already RNs, who complete a shorter course. During the course, students learn how to monitor the health of pregnant women, facilitate normal delivery and identify when extra assistance is needed. A significant proportion of training takes place in both a hospital and the community.

Health Visitor
Health Visitors (HVs) work with families to promote healthy lifestyles and teach parents how to keep children safe and well. Some HVs work with older people or at-risk groups, e.g. those with addiction problems or subject to domestic violence. HVs can work within GP practices, nurseries or schools. Strangely, they are managed (and paid) by local public health departments at the council – mainly as they were part of community and domiciliary care pillar in the 'original NHS' in 1948.

Day to day activities include:
- Antenatal and postnatal support to women
- Educating families on caring for their children
- Supporting children with disabilities
- Safeguarding.

Training
HVs must be a qualified nurse or midwife and will undertake an additional one-year training programme to qualify as a Specialist Community Public Health Nurse.

Paediatric Nurse
A paediatric, or children's, nurse will generally work with children aged up to 18 years (although there are exceptions), including new-born babies. This involves working in hospitals or the community. Maintaining the safety of young people is paramount and thus safeguarding is an important aspect of children's nursing.

Day-to-day activities include:
- Providing care to children who are ill
- Observing the condition of the child
- Administering medications
- Supporting parents/carers and communicating with them about a child's condition.

Training
The main route of training is via a three-year full time degree course at university, followed by registration with the NMC. Work experience such as volunteering or working in a nursery can give great insight. There are routes for adult RNs which allow them to train to work with children.

Mental Health Nurse
Mental health nurses work in psychiatric hospitals, prisons and the community to support patients with mental health problems. They specialise in working with different groups, such as children, the elderly, learning disability, drugs and alcohol or perinatal.

Day-to-day activities include:
- Building relationships with patients to allow them to talk openly
- Administering medication
- Encouraging patients and helping them take part in activities to improve their mental health.

Training
Training to become a mental health nurse requires a three-year university level degree, or apprenticeship, followed by registration with the NMC. Both routes require working alongside mental health nurses on psychiatric wards on placements. Volunteering with a mental health service or charity can provide useful insight before training.

Advanced Health Practitioner
Two relatively new groups of advanced health practitioners (AHPs) are becoming increasingly important in the NHS. They are designed to take on duties previously performed by doctors.

Physician Associate (PA)

Physician Associates (PAs) work under the supervision of doctors to support them in making diagnoses and treating patients. PAs can work independently from a doctor, but they will refer to a doctor if appropriate. This role can be within a hospital or GP practice.

Day-to-day activities include:
- Taking a history and doing an examination
- Ordering tests such as blood tests and analysing the results
- Making patient management plans
- Medical procedures such as cannulation.

PAs are not currently able to request imaging tests involving ionising radiation such as x-rays or CT scans. They are also not usually allowed to prescribe medication. However courses can be taken to train to be a prescriber.

Training

To train as a PA, an applicant will need to have a university degree in a bioscience related subject (including nursing or paramedicine), as this is usually a two-year graduate diploma or master's level course. There are some undergraduate courses now available with the possibility of apprenticeships in the future.

Training involves placements within a clinical setting and gaining theoretical knowledge through lectures. The PA role is not currently a regulated profession. There is, however, a Physician Associate Managed Voluntary Register to join on successful completion of the PA National Certifying Examination. It is hoped that the General Medical Council will regulate the profession soon. This role is not a route into becoming a doctor, with PAs needing to undertake to full training to attain this qualification.

Advanced Clinical Practitioner (ACP)

ACPs are healthcare professionals such as nurses, paramedics or pharmacists who are educated to master's level and have relevant experience contributing to a widened set of skills. ACPs can diagnose and treat certain conditions and refer patients. Within the NHS, ACPs can work within different specialties. This is a new role which is being developed and aims to better meet the health needs delivered by the multi-disciplinary team. Again, it is usually a two year course.

Doctor

The medical workforce continues to grow, with 121,700 doctors in the NHS in August 2020 including about 53,900 hospital consultants. From 2012 to 2020, the number of licensed doctors grew by more than 14%, including a record rise of 5% between 2019 and 2020. The UK medical workforce is increasingly ethnically diverse, with 54% of the doctors joining the register in 2020 identifying as black and minority ethnic (BAME). There are almost 10,000 doctors practicing registered aged over 70 in the UK.

As of December 2019, there were about 28,300 FTE GPs, a concerning 1% decrease from December 2018, and a 3% decrease from December 2017. There were 6,813 GP practices in England in February 2020, a decrease of 180 from February 2019. This means on average, more than three practices closed each week, although some of this reduction is due to smaller practices merging.

There are many different types of doctor, several of these are described below. All doctors who train in the UK must have a degree in medicine and complete the two-year UK Foundation Programme. They can then go on to specialise. The training pathway for doctors is complicated.

Medical School
There are currently 41 universities with medical schools in the UK. Many medical students enter straight from school after A levels, but there are other routes into training. It is important to research the entry criteria and options for medical school admission.

Different Types of Medical Course
Standard Entry. This is usually a five-year course, but it can be six. This results in the award of a 'Bachelor of Medicine and Bachelor of Surgery degree', with alternative abbreviations depending on the medical school.

Graduate Entry. This is a course open to those who hold a previous bachelor's degree usually with a minimum classification of a 2:1. It may be lower for those with a master's or PhD degree. Most universities require the first degree to be health/science related. As a result of already holding a degree, the course is normally 4 years of accelerated learning. Some medical schools (e.g. Warwick) only have a graduate entry course, and take any graduate, not just health/science.

Medicine with a Preliminary Year. This is the usual five-year course with an extra foundation year at the beginning. This year is normally for students who have achieved high scores at A level but not in science related subjects. The year is used for science learning.

Medicine with a Gateway Year. The usually five-year course has an extra year of training at the beginning. These courses are designed for those with high ability but where barriers exist to their learning, taking into account circumstances that may have made studying more difficult.

Medical Student Funding
For those on five- or six-year courses, a student loan can be obtained from Student Finance England, who will fund tuition fees and living expenses. In year 5 onwards, the NHS Student Bursary Team fund tuition fees and living expenses. Funding for those who already have a degree and enter a five-year standard entry is different, with no tuition fee grants available. Maintenance loans may however be available. During the final year of medical school, NHS Bursary funding is available. Recently, private medical schools have opened in the UK.

Graduate Funding. This is different, with £3,465 of first year tuition fees being self-funded, and Student Finance funding £3,465. After this, NHS Bursaries fund £3,465 each year with Student Finance covering the remainder of the tuition fees.

Entry Requirements
Entry Exams. Entry into medical school does not just focus on academic grades. Different medical schools use different tests for entry. Most UK universities use the UCAT (University Clinical Aptitude test), while a few apply the BMAT (Biomedical Admissions Test). Some graduate routes use the GAMSAT (Graduate Australian Medical School Admission Test).

Work Experience. Medical schools often require evidence of work experience which may involve observing doctors in practice. More important is experience and reflection on caring roles, as these demonstrate key qualities needed to be a doctor, e.g. volunteering in a care home, hospital or disability care setting.

Interview. Medical schools will usually require an interview to gain a place. Interview types include panel interviews of up to three people, and multiple mini-interviews involving a number of stations. Assessment centre interviews involve different tasks and can include group activities and written work. Contacting each medical school and finding out their interview format can be helpful.

Foundation Training
After graduation, doctors are provisionally licenced to practise with the GMC, which allows individuals to join the UK Foundation Programme; a 2-year rotational programme (of six 4-month blocks) within a defined geographical region known as a 'Deanery'. After successful completion of the first year, full registration with GMC is granted, which allows the doctor to practice as an independent prescriber. Foundation training is paid and takes place within a hospital, with the opportunity to rotate into general practice.

General Practitioner
GPs work in 'surgeries' and treat common conditions that do not require hospital admissions. If a GP feels a patient needs more complex assessment or treatment, they can refer them to a specialist doctor, either in secondary or tertiary care. They are often considered the backbone of the NHS.

Some GPs have a 'special interest' – where they undertake further training to become 'specialised' in an area of medicine whilst also being a GP, e.g. mental health, paediatrics or obstetrics and gynaecology. In the UK's traditional model of general practice, a GP can choose to be a 'partner' which means they own the building and oversee the running of their own practice. Being a non-partner GP is increasingly popular; including 'salaried', 'portfolio' or 'locum' GPs.

Day-to-day activities for a GP include:
- Consultations - either face to face or via telephone - with patients. These typically last 10 minutes
- Prescribing medication
- Interpreting blood tests
- Administration duties such as signing 'Fitness to Work' notes and writing referrals for patients who need more specialist input or urgent treatment.

Training
Upon completing the two years of Foundation Training, a doctor wishing to be a GP will apply to a 3-year Specialist GP training course. This usually includes 18 months working within a hospital on different four to six month 'rotations' (e.g. Gynaecology, Paediatrics), and a further 18 months within a GP practice. To work as a GP, doctors must join the GMC's GP Register.

Hospital Physician

The largest area of hospital medicine that is not surgery (and everything else) is confusingly called 'medicine'. In the past it was called 'general medicine' and, in the USA, 'internal medicine'. The doctors who practice it are called *physicians*. There are many medical specialties including: cardiology, respiratory medicine, gastroenterology, diabetes and endocrinology, rheumatology, dermatology, geriatric medicine, acute medicine, nephrology, haematology and oncology. Medical doctors may work on wards, in outpatient clinics, perform procedures, take part in multidisciplinary team meetings - and undertake research, administration and teaching.

Training
After completing the Foundation Programme, trainees can apply to the 2-3 year Internal Medicine Training (IMT) programme (previously called Core Medical Training, or CMT). This is formed from two groups of medical specialties. These are: Group 1 Specialties (e.g. cardiology), which are the specialties most likely to provide acute care in the hospital; and Group 2 Specialties, which are specialties that mainly provide non-acute outpatient services (e.g. oncology).

Doctors who want to become a consultant in a Group 1 Specialty, must do all three years of the IMT programme. After completion, they can apply for a position in their preferred specialty, to continue in 'Specialty and Internal Medicine training'. This is approximately four years long but can vary by specialty and is often called the 'registrar' period. These trainees must undertake a further 12 months of internal (general) medicine training as part of their Stage 2 training (i.e. they must do a more 'general year' as part of the four years).

Doctors that wish to become a Consultant in a Group 2 Specialty, complete two of the three years of IMT. After completing their second year, trainees are eligible to take up specialty training in their chosen specialty. Specialty Training is approximately four years long.

A full list of Group 1 and Group 2 specialties can be found on the Joint Royal Colleges of Physicians Training Board website.

Those wishing to specialise in certain specialties including Emergency Medicine can alternatively complete the 'Acute Care Common Stem' training programme, which is three years long, and occurs after the two years of the Foundation Programme.

Upon completion of specialty training in all these areas, trainees are eligible to apply for a consultant post.

Surgeon

Surgical doctors operate on patients in operating theatres. The work of a surgeon is varied, as they also spend time doing ward rounds, outpatient clinics, procedures (like colonoscopy), research, teaching and administration.

Surgeons choose a speciality to work within, each of which vary in terms of how competitive they are to gain a place on the training programme. There are 10 main surgical specialties, many of which are made up of sub-specialties. These are: general surgery, neurosurgery, cardiothoracic surgery, paediatric surgery, urology, plastic surgery, otolaryngology (known as ENT), oral and maxillofacial surgery, trauma and orthopaedic surgery, and vascular surgery.

Training

After the 2-year 'foundation programme', those wishing to become surgeons may either apply to Core Surgical Training (CST), or directly to Specialty Training (ST - only available for certain surgical specialties). Core surgical training is a two year rotational programme, where trainees spend four 6-month blocks in different surgical specialties.

Specialty training (as a 'registrar') in surgery is approximately six years long (though many do extra years to gain very specialist skills); and upon completion, trainees are allowed to register on the GMC's Specialist Register. Once completed, individuals can apply for consultant posts.

Radiologist

Radiologists are doctors who diagnose, monitor and treat patients using different types of medical images and provide specialist input at multidisciplinary team meetings. Radiologists have the option to specialise in a particular area of radiology (e.g. musculoskeletal radiology or neuroradiology; the latter focus on CTs and MRIs of the spine and brain) or work as generalists.

There are a wide variety of techniques used for medical imaging, including: x-ray, ultrasound, magnetic resonance imaging (MRI), computed tomography (CT), nuclear medicine and positron emission tomography (PET).

Medical imaging has allowed procedures to be developed which are less invasive (than surgery) with 'Interventional Radiologists' performing such techniques including: angiography/angioplasty/stent insertion, biopsy, oesophageal stenting, biliary drainage and stenting. Many of these techniques have replaced traditional invasive operations.

Training

To become a radiologist, the applicant needs to have a degree in Medicine and have completed the 2-year Foundation Programme. Following on from this, they enter Specialty

Training (ST) for radiology which takes five years to complete, with five stages taking the trainee from 'ST1' to 'ST5'. Three of these years are spent training in general radiology and the final two years are spent learning an area of specialist interest. Trainees can complete an additional 'ST6 year' to train in interventional radiology. After completion of the training programme, trainees may apply for a consultant post.

Psychiatrist

A psychiatrist is a medical doctor who specialises in mental health. Psychiatrists diagnose and manage psychiatric conditions such as depression, anxiety, schizophrenia, dementia and eating disorders. Psychiatrists work on inpatient psychiatric wards, in outpatient clinics and the community.

Day-to-day activities include:
- Assessing a patient's mental health, and deciding if they are a risk to themselves or others
- Prescribing medications and deciding which other therapies a patient may need (a wide range, from talking therapies to electroconvulsive therapy)
- There are several subspecialities in psychiatry:
    - Child and adolescent: patients aged 18 years and under
    - Perinatal psychiatry: psychiatric disorders occur in the perinatal period
    - Forensic: patients in prison or secure hospitals
    - Old age: patients over 65 years with illnesses such as dementia
    - Medical psychotherapy: using psychotherapy to help treat mental illnesses.

Training
After deciding to pursue training in psychiatry, three years of 'core training' is undertaken following the foundation years. After this, there is 'higher training' (registrar) lasting three years. Upon completion, a trainee can apply to be a consultant.

Clinical Psychologist

Clinical psychologists are different from psychiatrists. They are not (usually) medically trained doctors but have studied clinical psychology. Psychologists provide support to those with mental illness, including those suffering with addiction or trauma. Part of the job involves assessing a patient's state of mind and working in partnership with them to manage their mental health. Training in specific therapies such as Cognitive Behavioural Therapy (CBT) can lead to teaching these techniques to patients. Clinical Psychology is varied and can involve working with adults or children, in hospitals, clinics or Improving Access to Psychological Therapies (IAPT) services.

Training
After studying for a psychology degree at university, postgraduate professional training is required. This is either a 2-year postgraduate qualification, or two years of supervised experience with a registered psychologist.

Psychiatrists may undertake further training to become a psychologist, and are therefore able to specialise in 'talking therapy' in addition to the prescribing of 'psychotropic' medication.

Independent Doctor

Following full registration with the GMC (after completing foundation year one), a doctor may technically leave foundation training and practice as an independent doctor, within or outside of the NHS. If they wish to later pursue a GMC-approved training programme, they must re-enter and complete their FY2 year. Most go on to finish the two years. Others may choose not to go into training after finishing the two years of the foundation programme but continue to work as a doctor. Independent doctors may privately prescribe most medicines and carry out some procedures (after an accredited training course), e.g. Botox - if they hold full GMC registration.

Independent non-specialist doctors, however, may not prescribe certain medications like chemotherapy, or perform most types of surgery. It is difficult to become a GP or consultant (a specialist) in the UK without formal training. There are however new training pathways such as CESR (Certificate of Eligibility for Specialist Registration) that allows trainees to submit a portfolio of evidence for consideration and apply for a consultant post, without completing a GMC-approved training programme.

Summary

Figure 4.2 summarises current medical training in the UK.

Dentist

Dentists provide care for patients' mouths and teeth. They can also be involved in treating dental and facial injuries. In the UK, there were over 39,000 dentists in 12,100 practices in 2017. Though it is of concern that 23,733 dentists performed NHS activity in England during 2020-21, a decrease of 951 on the previous year.

Much of a dentist's work centres on preventing tooth decay and oral disease. They oversee the wider dental team within primary care. Practices are either private, NHS or a mix of both, as well as providing services within hospitals. Most dentists are General Dental Practitioners (GDPs).

Day-to-day activities include:
- Examining mouths and teeth, and performing investigations, e.g. x-rays, and providing treatment
- Education regarding oral hygiene and disease prevention.

About 15% of dentists own the surgery where they work, while salaried dentists work for the practice owners. There has been a growth of corporate ownership of dental practices with 'Mydentist' being the biggest in the UK, with over 650 practices and 3,000 dentists.

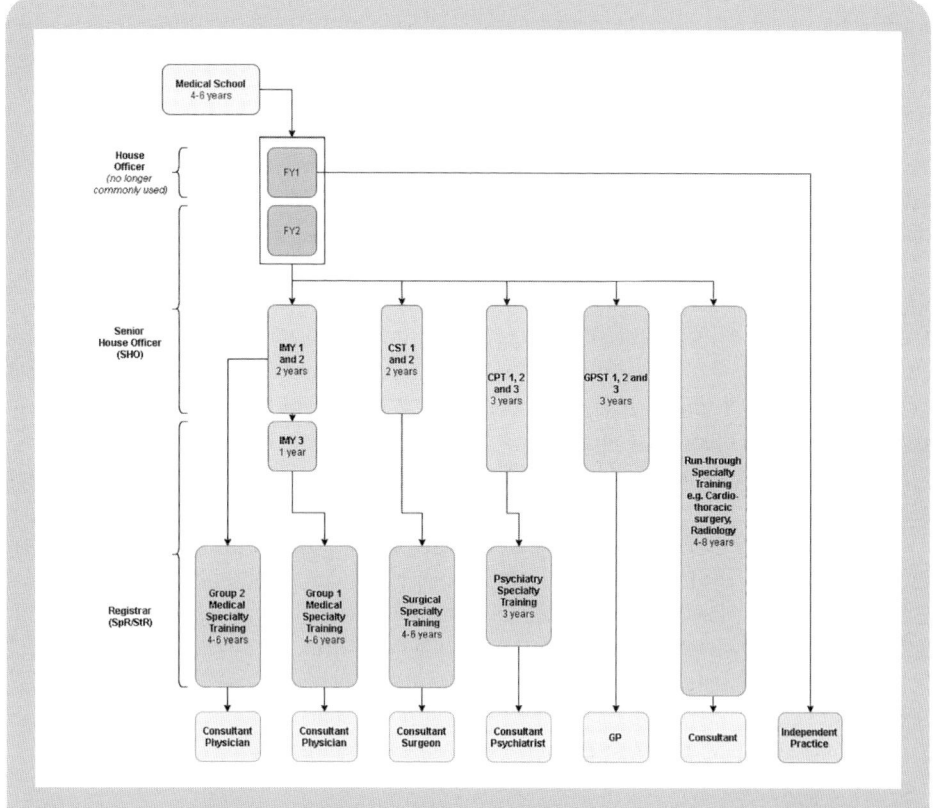

Figure 4.2: A non-exhaustive diagram of training pathways to full qualification for different types of doctors in the UK.

Training

Most entrants require a minimum of three As at A-level, although 1-year pre-dental courses are offered by some dental schools. Those with a 2:1 bachelor's degree in a science or biomedical subject can apply to a small number of 4-year graduate entry courses allowing direct entry to the 2nd year (or combine the curriculum of years 1 and 2 into a single year).

Becoming a dentist is like medical training, with five years of undergraduate study, but one (not two) year of Foundation Training. This is only a requirement for dentists who wish to enter the NHS Performers List and work as an NHS dentist. Unlike for doctors, following undergraduate study, a dental graduate can work privately without completing the 1-year Foundation Training. All UK dentists must be registered with the General Dental Council.

After foundation training, a dentist may opt to undergo non-compulsory Dental Core Training (DCT) that has multiple endpoints and varies from one to three years. This training programme is designed to supplement a dentist's skillsets. After this, most GDPs work within a general practice, performing NHS and private work. If a dentist decides to perform only private work, then they can earn more, but lose NHS benefits such as the NHS pension and maternity/paternity pay.

Dentists can sub-specialise in 13 areas recognised by the General Dental Council, including orthodontics and dental public health. To do this, they need to become a registrar after core training, and undertake Specialty Training (usually three years of full-time, paid training).

Dental Nurse

Dental nurses are GDC-registered and provide clinical and other support to GDPs and patients. Trainee dental nurses do not need any academic qualifications. Qualified dental nurses' study, either part or full time, undertaking a General Dental Council approved course. Part-time course requirements vary between providers, but a minimum 2 GCSEs (4/C grade or above) in English language and mathematics, or a science subject, are usually needed.

Full-time degree level courses may require A-levels, or equivalent level 3 qualifications. A level 3 apprenticeship in dental nursing is also available. With extra training, a dental nurse can take x-rays and clinical photographs, take impressions, make models of teeth, and apply fluoride varnish to prevent tooth decay. With experience, they can train to be a dental hygienist, dental or orthodontic therapist. A nurse can also acquire additional skills such as impression-taking and providing fluoride varnish as part of a dental public health programme.

Dental Hygienist

Dental hygienists are GDC-registered and help patients maintain their oral health by preventing and treating periodontal disease and promoting good oral health practice. They carry out treatment direct to patients or under prescription from a dentist.

Dental Therapist

Dental therapists are GDC-registered dental professionals who carry out dental treatments direct to patients or under prescription from a dentist. Therapists offer a wider range of treatments than Hygienists.

Allied Health Professionals

Allied Health Professionals (AHPs) are involved in the delivery of day-to-day patient care. The majority of AHPs are degree-level and are regulated by the Health and Care Professions Council (HCPC), except Osteopaths. This group of health professionals will now be described.

Dietitian

Dietitians diagnose and treat nutritional problems and help modify diets to manage health. They give advice on nutrition and dietary problems, and can work in hospitals or the community. Dietitians may work with people that:
- Want to lose weight
- Have a food allergy/intolerance

- Have an eating disorder
- Have a long-term condition and need adequate nutrition (e.g. diabetes).

Day-to-day activities include:
- Undertaking nutritional assessments
- Educating and advising patients on ways to improve their diet
- Creating nutritional care plans and monitoring their efficacy.

Training
There are 3-year university dietetic courses at undergraduate level and 2-year at postgraduate level. Courses involve both clinical placements and theory. Many qualified dietitians will register with the British Dietetic Association as well as the HCPC. This allows dietitians to ensure their practice is up to date. Dietitians may work outside of the NHS (e.g. in sports nutrition or the food industry), where working hours and pay will differ.

Physiotherapist

The role of a physiotherapist is to improve patients' quality of life by increasing their functional ability and mobility. This means working with people of all ages; usually seeing people with injuries, disability or illness. Physiotherapists can specialise in a range of areas, e.g. musculoskeletal, stroke, sporting injury, or cardiac rehabilitation.

Physiotherapists can work in many different environments including hospitals, fitness centres, in patients' homes, GP practices or care homes.

Day-to-day work includes:
- Implementing programmes to improve patients' physical functioning
- Giving health advice to patients
- Preventing functional deterioration in patients.

Training
An undergraduate or postgraduate degree - either as part of a university course or whilst employed as an apprentice - must be completed to become a physiotherapist. Undergraduate programmes are usually three years. Whereas postgraduate courses are normally two years, and degree apprenticeship programmes typically last four years. As well as registering with the HCPC, physiotherapists can register with the Chartered Society of Physiotherapy, which offers professional support and training and development opportunities.

Occupational Therapist

Occupational therapists (OTs) work with patients to overcome functional barriers and improve their quality of life. This empowers patients towards achieving their full potential, and complete activities and day-to-day as independently as possible. OTs work with people from all ages including those with a diagnosis of a learning or physical disability, or a mental health condition.

Day-to-day working includes:
- Identifying functional barriers to activity (and making plans to overcome these)
- Encouraging patients to explore new activities
- Helping people to live independently.

Training
All OTs are required to complete a degree that is accredited by the Royal College of Occupational Therapists. Most of these courses are undergraduate degrees, but postgraduate ones are available. The degree can also be completed through an apprenticeship course, which is a combination of academic teaching and work placements.

Speech and Language Therapist

Speech and language therapists (SALT/SLTs) specialise in working with people who have difficulties in swallowing, eating, drinking and/or communicating. They look after people with a wide variety of conditions, e.g. dementia and learning difficulties. SLTs work with people of all ages in highly varied environments within the NHS, including schools, children's centres, clients' homes, prisons - or within private practice.

Training
SLTs are required to have completed a degree-level course accredited by the Royal College of Speech and Language Therapists (RCSLT) and approved by the HCPC. There are SLT programmes for both undergraduate, typically 2-4 years, and postgraduate (MSc or PGDip) students, typically two years.

The RCSLT are establishing a new 4-year, paid degree apprenticeship training programme for SLTs, where trainees apply directly to an employer who is linked to an accredited university.

Radiographer

Radiographers use different types of imaging technology to obtain images of the inside of peoples' bodies which are used to diagnose and monitor disease. Imaging technology includes x-rays, CT (computed tomography), MRI (magnetic resonance imaging), fluoroscopy and ultrasound.

Day-to-day tasks include:
- Undertaking radiographic images of patients
- Assisting in complex radiological procedures with radiologists (doctors).

Training
All radiographers must complete an approved full-time undergraduate degree (3-4 years), or a postgraduate course (typically two years). There are some apprenticeship degree courses.

Therapeutic Radiographer

Therapeutic radiographers (or, radiotherapists) usually work with cancer patients and provide treatments, such as ionising radiation, to patients. Therapeutic radiographers work with clinical radiographers (and clinical oncologists, i.e. doctors) to design treatment plans, and ensure tumours receive the right dose of radiation whilst minimising harm to surrounding tissues. Training involves a 3-4 year undergraduate degree or a master's degree in radiotherapy.

Operating Department Practitioner

Operating department practitioners (ODPs) mainly work within operating theatres and may be involved in surgery, anaesthetics or recovery.

Day-to-day roles in surgery include:
- Being part of the surgical team (they may be 'scrubbed')
- Being responsible for all equipment within the theatre.

Day-to-day roles in anaesthetics include:
- Ensuring that anaesthetic equipment is working correctly
- Ensuring all anaesthetic drugs required, are available
- Assisting the anaesthetist in the induction of anaesthesia and throughout the procedure.

Day-to-day roles in recovery include:
- Providing appropriate treatment to the patient to help in their recovery from surgery
- Assessing when the patient is ready to be transferred to a ward.

Training
ODP students can either complete a 3-year degree or a 2-year diploma at university. Degree apprenticeship programmes are being introduced, where students are employed within an organisation that is linked to an education provider (and complete the 3-year degree).

Podiatrist

Podiatrists are healthcare professionals who are trained to diagnose and manage abnormal conditions of the lower limbs and feet. They help prevent and correct deformity, improve mobility and treat infections as well as offering useful lifestyle advice including on foot ware. They work mainly outside of the NHS but can provide NHS care for certain patients, e.g. those with diabetes.

Pharmacist

Pharmacists are specialists in medication, and have a detailed understanding of medication safety, medication interactions, side effects, recommended doses, and the form in which they should be prescribed (e.g. tablet or injection). They also provide advice directly to patients or other healthcare professionals. Pharmacists also provide specialist health advice including information about smoking cessation and sexual health. Some pharmacists prescribe medication following the completion of a prescribing course.

Pharmacists work in hospitals, community settings, primary care, universities or the pharmaceutical industry.

Training
Pharmacists must complete a master's degree in pharmacy (MPharm), usually 4-years fulltime, accredited by the General Pharmaceutical Council (GPhC). To be eligible, students normally require science A levels at grades A-B, or must complete a pharmacy foundation degree. Pharmacists complete a pre-registration training period of 12 months before they can be registered as a pharmacist with the GPhC.

Pharmacy Technician
Pharmacy technicians assist pharmacists. They manage and prepare the supply of medicines and give advice to patients and customers. In a community pharmacy, pharmacy technicians may be involved in delivering some public health services such as advice on stopping smoking.

Training
Pharmacy technicians require an accredited qualification such as: BTEC National Diploma in pharmaceutical science, NVQ/SVQ level 3 in pharmacy services, or National Certificate in pharmaceutical science. To apply for a course, they need to be working in a pharmacy. Employers, including the NHS, offer jobs for trainee pharmacy technicians. Pharmacy technicians must be registered with the GPhC.

Paramedics and Other Ambulance Staff
Calls to 999 are often responded to by paramedics, meaning they often deal with life-threatening illness. However, they also deal with minor injuries and non-emergency situations. Paramedics usually work in pairs, but they also work alone in emergency response cars.

Day-to-day activities include:
- Assessing a patient's condition and deciding if they require hospital treatment
- Managing emergency care provision
- Working with other emergency services such as police, firefighters and coast guards.

Paramedics work closely with healthcare professionals in EDs and some now work for GPs, carrying out home visits; as well as in hospices where they may be involved in prescribing pain relief and similar medications.

Training
Paramedics must complete an HCPC-approved qualification usually at university on a 3-year BSc degree. Some courses also require paramedics to hold a full, or provisional, UK C1 driving licence. Paramedic apprenticeships are often paid positions which offer 'on

the job' training working as an ambulance technician. Experience in a caring position is helpful and some of the roles described below can provide a good foundation for further training as a paramedic.

Ambulance Technician. Ambulance technicians work supporting paramedics but may also work alone responding to 999 calls. Technicians can progress to team leader or apply to train as a paramedic.

Emergency Care Assistant

They work under the direction and supervision of paramedics when responding to emergencies. Roles include:

- Checking equipment on the ambulance
- Keeping patients calm
- Providing first aid
- Treating wounds.

Patient Transport Service

PTS staff assist and drive disabled, vulnerable or elderly patients to and from hospital appointments or admission.

Call Handler

Call handlers answer 999 calls and gather important information about a patient's condition and location. They assist with emergencies via the telephone and provide instructions to the caller, including how best to provide first aid.

Manager

The introduction of (General) Managers (GMs) into the NHS followed the publication of the Griffiths Report in 1983. There is a famous quote in the report which says that if Florence Nightingale were walking the hospital corridors with her lamp, she would struggle to find the person in charge. The report also recommended doctors should take a stronger role in managing health and hospitals.

There is a 2-year (2.5 years if specialising in finance) NHS Graduate Management Training Scheme. There are several specialist pathways: Finance, General Management, Health Analysis, Health Informatics, Human Resources, Policy and Strategy. People from other NHS roles (e.g. nurse, AHP or porter) can (and do) climb the management ladder, without undertaking the graduate programme.

Hospital Management Structure

Hospital management is hierarchical, usually with three 'levels': Departmental, Divisional (or Directorate) and Executive. At each level there is a triumvirate of Clinical Director (usually a Doctor), Nurse and Manager 'in charge'. It is important that one person is responsible and accountable for the running of a Department or Division. This is usually the Clinical Director (any suitable healthcare professional), i.e. retaining the importance of clinical leadership.

Hospital Clinical Manager

These managers oversee a Department (or Division, i.e. group of Departments, like Surgical or Medical) within a hospital, leading a team of healthcare professionals; and may be an NHS-trained manager, or other qualified professional. They plan for the needs of a Department (or Division) and set its priorities and targets; as well as being responsible for clinical audits, governance, mandatory training, among other roles.

Human Resources (HR)

HR are responsible for staff recruitment, training and appraisals. There are many roles within HR, but all support frontline staff to enable care delivery.

Hospital Senior Manager

The most senior managers are called Executive Directors (or 'Executives'), with most being on the Trust Board. In NHS hospitals there are two senior managers (Chief Executive and Chief Operating Officer) who work with a doctor (Chief Medical Officer), a nurse (Chief Nursing Officer) and a Chief Financial Officer (and sometimes a head of strategy).

Executive Directors and Trust (or Organisation) Board

Chief Executive Officer (CEO)
This is the operational head who manages the services and business of the Trust and implements the decisions of the Trust Board. Many will have started as a junior hospital manager; some are doctors or nurses. When CEOs are appointed, they sign a document presented by the Secretary of State which sets out their responsibilities and accountabilities as CEO; this formally appoints them as the 'Accountable Officer'.

Chief Operating Officer (COO)
The COO is usually responsible for the day-to-day operation of the hospital, implementing board strategy as well as emergency planning and response. In most hospitals, they also manage the estate and facilities. Clinical Directors usually report to the COO because their services are at the heart of the hospitals function.

Medical Director (MD: also called Chief Medical Officer, CMO)
The CMO is a senior doctor who is an advocate for patients at Board level. They are crucial in driving up the standards of care, clinical safety and governance, and communicating with staff on the front-line.

Chief Nursing Officer (CNO)
The CNO is responsible for all things related to nursing, including strategy, and usually for the AHPs.

Chief Financial Officer (CFO)
The CFO is responsible for financial management.

Staff and Training

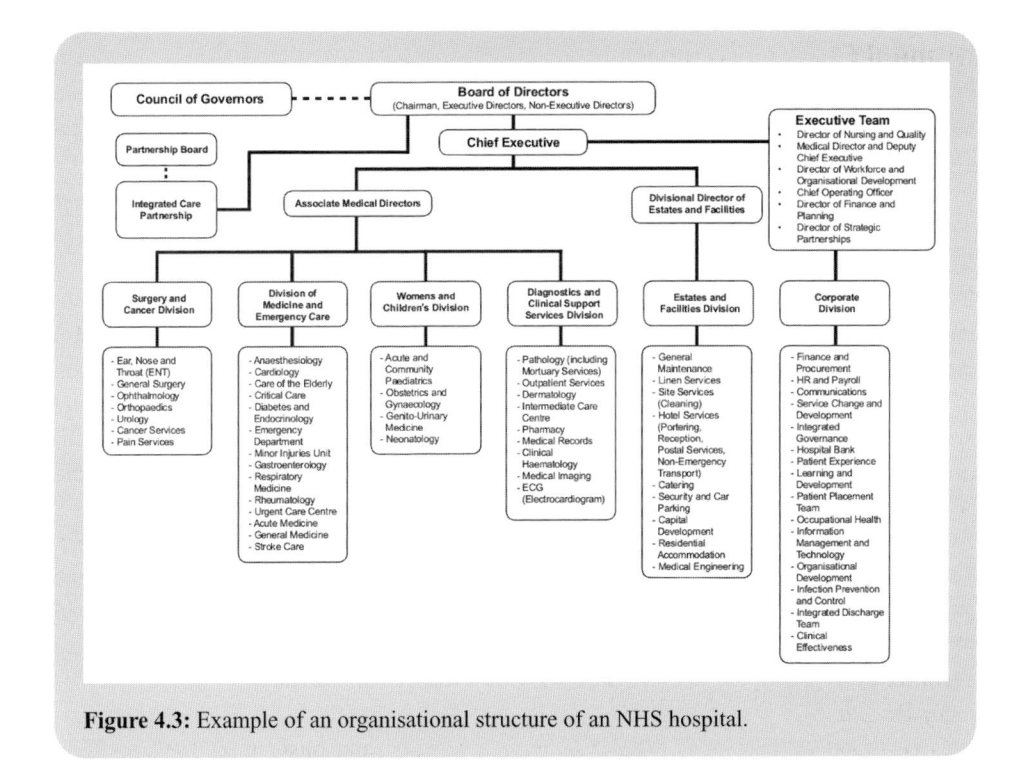

Figure 4.3: Example of an organisational structure of an NHS hospital.

Trust Board, Chairperson and Non-Executive Directors (NEDs)
NHS Trust Boards are 'unitary', i.e. they have collective responsibility for all the work of the Trust. This is quite complex as the NEDs (who come from a range of backgrounds) are both part of the Board, but also have responsibility for the public interest, by holding the Executive Directors, including the CEO, to account. They are employed by the Trust/organisation to be independent and promote high standards as well as leading effective decision-making processes. Both the Chairperson and CEO have statutory responsibilities, including for things that go wrong in the Trust. The Chair and other non-executives can hire and fire the CEO.

The Board will have several different sub-committees that focus on managing individual aspects of the organisation including Finance and Performance, Quality and Workforce.

Summary of Hospital Structure
Figure 4. 3 is an example of the management structure of a large hospital.

Other Managers

NHS England and CCGs
The NHS's administration system - including CCGs and NHS England - are mainly staffed by managers, many of whom will have worked in hospitals or other clinical settings.

Practice Manager
Practice managers are involved with managing the business aspects of the GP surgery and ensure accurate record keeping and good administration occurs.

Other Roles

Biomedical Scientist (or Medical Laboratory Scientific Officer, MLSO)
Biomedical scientists work in medical laboratories and use scientific techniques to interpret information from patients by analysing tissue samples and fluids. They aid the diagnosis, monitoring and the treatment of disease. They can monitor the condition of patients, e.g. by assessing kidney function, or can ensure correct blood products are available in emergencies. Biomedical scientists usually specialise in blood, infection or cellular sciences.

Training
To qualify as a biomedical scientist, registered with the HCPC, individuals must complete an Institute of Biomedical Sciences Accredited Degree Programme at undergraduate or postgraduate level. Those who have undertaken a non-accredited biomedical science degree, can have their degree assessed and may be required to complete top-up modules to qualify.

Further reading

House of Commons briefing on the key statistics, including staffing in the NHS.

https://researchbriefings.files.parliament.uk/documents/CBP-7281/CBP-7281.pdf

A King's Fund overview of staffing in the NHS.

https://www.kingsfund.org.uk/projects/nhs-in-a-nutshell/nhs-workforce

An NHS page about careers in the NHS.

https://www.healthcareers.nhs.uk/explore-roles

Chapter 5

Organisations

"Teamwork is the ability to work together toward a common vision... and organizational objectives. It is the fuel that allows common people to attain uncommon results." Andrew Carnegie (1835-1919).

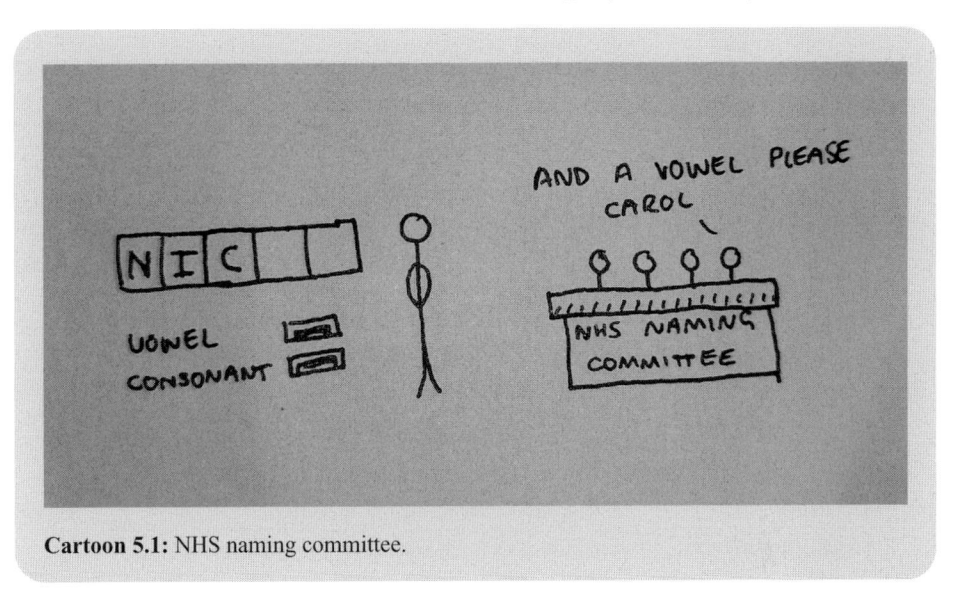

Cartoon 5.1: NHS naming committee.

Background

This quote is true for all large systems, including healthcare ones which require multiple organisations to run them. This chapter describes these organisations and how they fit together to form the complicated and confusing thing we call the NHS.

Although the NHS has made great strides in enhancing healthcare, there remain many challenges including an ageing and growing population, evolving health needs, cost of novel medication and medical technology, staff training and recruitment.

This chapter will introduce the key organisations within the NHS, highlighting their roles and importance in empowering both professionals and the public to take ownership of their NHS - and work collaboratively to develop, change and improve the delivery of care.

Figure 5.1 summarises the current structure of the NHS in England unless otherwise stated. The rest of the chapter identifies what these organisations do.

Level	Health	Other
UK Administration (Government Department)	Department of Health and Social Care (England only); NHS Scotland, NHS Wales and NHS Northern Ireland	Department for Levelling Up, Housing and Communities. (Local Government) or other departments
National Administration	NHS England (NHSE)	
National Public Health (PH)	Public Health England (being replaced by UK Health Security Agency, HSA), PH Scotland, PH Wales, PH Agency (NI)	
Other National Linked Bodies (linked to NHSE)	NHS Digital/X, Health Research Authority, NHS Blood and Transplant, Medicines and Healthcare Products Regulatory Agency, NHS Business Services Authority, NHS Resolution, Human Fertilisation and Embryology Authority, Human Tissue Authority, NHS Counter Fraud Authority	Healthwatch England Local Healthwatch
Commissioners / Other	CCG, NHS Regions (Specialist Commissioning), ICS (combining CCGs and Healthcare Delivery)	Local Health & Well-being Board
Healthcare Delivery	Primary Care/Primary Care Networks (PCNs), Secondary Care, Community/Other Care, Prisons	Local PH Social Care Armed Services (MoD)
Regulatory and Monitoring	NICE, CQC, Dr Foster, Professional Councils (GMC, NMC etc)	
Education and Training	HEE, LTEBs, Royal Colleges and Professional Bodies, Universities	
Other	Charities, Think Tanks, Royal Society Medicine, Unions	

Figure 5.1: Summary of NHS Structure (England unless stated).

National Leadership - Department of Health and Social Care (DHSC)

The Government of the United Kingdom exercises executive authority through two main types of 'Government Departments': Ministerial and Non-ministerial. The DHSC is one out of a total of 24 ministerial departments. It was created in 1988 and was previously known as the Ministry of Health and Department of Health ('DH') amongst other names.

The DHSC sets the overall policy on all issues, including public health and the health consequences of environmental and food issues. It is also responsible for the provision of healthcare via hospitals, semi-independent contractors such as GPs, dentists, pharmacists, opticians, and other organisations. Its primary purpose is to improve the health and wellbeing of people in UK. The DHSC is supported by, and works through, 29 agencies of three main types: Executive agencies, Executive non-departmental public bodies, and Advisory non-departmental public bodies.

The idea is that they are linked to DHSC without being run by them, so they can be run by professionals, with a degree of independence. In fact, NHS England (NHSE, which 'runs' healthcare in England) is one such body (a very large one), that takes most of the DHSC budget. None of these bodies are totally free of government scrutiny, which in a democracy, is right and proper.

The DHSC is accountable to parliament for health and adult social care and is led by the Secretary of State for Health and Social Care (HSC). The Secretary of State is supported by three ministers of state and two Parliamentary under-secretaries of state.

Commissioning

Commissioning is the process of ensuring health and care services are provided effectively and meet the needs of the population. At a simple level, it means buying healthcare. But commissioning is an extensive process, which requires assessing the needs of the local population, deciding priorities and strategies, planning service delivery, purchasing services and monitoring and evaluating delivery.

Before the 1990s, there was no separation between commissioning and the 'providing' role, e.g. hospital services. But the NHS and Community Care Act in 1990 created a split between the 'purchasing role' (which remained with health authorities) and the 'providing role' (which became the responsibility of newly formed NHS trusts, GPs, and other groups). The idea was to create an 'internal market' where providers would compete for resources thereby ensuring greater efficiency, responsiveness, and innovation - and the better providers would thrive.

Today, in England, the NHS commissioning bodies who carry out the purchasing role include:
- Clinical Commissioning Groups
- NHS England (including Specialist Commissioning).

Local Commissioning - Clinical Commissioning Groups (CCGs)

CCGs were established in April 2013, as part of the Health and Social Care Act (HSC Act) 2012 and took over the duties of the Primary Care Trusts commissioning of up to two-thirds of the NHS Budget. As of April 2020, there were 135 CCGs in England each serving around 250,000 people.

CCGs are independent bodies made up of groups of GP practices, with all GP practices in England being legally obliged to be members. They are led by an elected governing board of at least six professionals – an accountable officer, finance officer, registered nurse, secondary care specialist and two lay members. The health services commissioned by CCGs include:
- Urgent and Emergency Care
- Elective Hospital Care
- Community Health
- Rehabilitation
- Maternity and New-born

- Children Healthcare
- Services for People with Learning Disabilities
- Mental Health
- Infertility
- NHS Continuing Healthcare.

CCGs can commission services from a range of providers including voluntary and private sector providers. All providers must be legally registered with a monitoring or regulatory body. CCGs are accountable to NHSE for their performance.

To achieve successfull commissioning of services, CCGs collaborate with multiple organisations on a national, regional, and local level. These are some organisations which support CCGs:
- **Commissioning Support Units (CSU).** There are nine CSUs in England providing a range of 'backroom' services, e.g. contract management and negotiation, information and data analysis, and service redesign.
- **Strategic Clinical Networks.** These focus on key areas of priority within healthcare to reduce unwanted variation in services and encourage innovation.
- **Clinical Senates.** The 10 clinical senates in England are advisory groups, established to provide independent, strategic advice and guidance to commissioners.

Health and Wellbeing Boards

Health and Wellbeing Boards (HWBs), established in April 2013 as part of the HSC Act 2012, are committees created by local authorities to oversee commissioning and the co-ordination of HSC services. They aim to promote greater local integration and partnership and reduce health inequalities.

HWBs bring together bodies from the NHS, public health and local government including 'Healthwatch' (see below). HWBs produce a yearly Joint Strategic Needs Assessment (JSNA), which identifies the present and future health and care needs of local populations.

Subregional Commissioning - Sustainability and Transformation Partnership/ Integrated Care System (STP/ICS)

As part of the 2014 NHS *Five Year Forward View*, 44 Sustainability and Transformation Partnerships (STPs) were set up, one for each area of England of over one million people. They were voluntary, informal groupings of different NHS Trusts. Most are evolving into tighter groups called Integrated Care Systems (ICSs).

In August 2021, most STPs were on their way to form the final target of 42 ICSs. When their function is legalised, they may be given responsibility for workforce, commissioning, finances and waiting lists.

National Commissioning – NHS England

NHS England (NHSE) was established in April 2013 as part of the HSC Act 2012. It was initially named the NHS Commissioning Board Authority, which is still its statutory name.

It is an independent clinically led organisation which aims to improve health outcomes and deliver high quality care. Its responsibilities are discharged through seven regional teams and include:
- Overseeing the operations of CCGs
- Allocation of funds and resources to CCGs
- Direct commissioning of certain services including:
  - Primary care (GP, dentistry, optometry)
  - Community pharmacies
  - Provision of national leadership and guidance on commissioning
  - Health services for people in prisons and other custodial settings
  - Health services for members of the armed forces.

In 2018 it was announced, while maintaining its statutory independence, NHSE would be merged with NHS Improvement, and establish seven 'single integrated regional teams'.

National/Regional Commissioning - Specialist Commissioning
There is a separate system for commissioning specialist healthcare from the budgets of the NHSE regions. This system is for rare and expensive diseases, where a clinical service is not needed in every hospital, e.g. dialysis, transplantation, cardiac and neurosurgery and cancer care. Up to 30% of the income of large teaching hospitals comes via specialist commissioning.

Monitoring and Regulatory Bodies
Monitoring is the systematic process of observing and collecting data to assess if projects are being implemented as planned and if changes are needed. Given its size, monitoring in the NHS is crucial.

Healthwatch England
Healthwatch England was established in April 2013, as part of the HSC Act 2012, and is the national independent consumer champion for HSC. It exists at a national level (Healthwatch England) and at a local level (Local Healthwatch). The primary aim of Local Healthwatch is to understand the needs, experiences and concerns of local people and make these known to local authorities, providers and commissioners. Healthwatch England provides national leadership for the local Healthwatch networks.

NHS Improvement (NHSI)[10]
NHSI was the operational name for several different bodies responsible for overseeing foundation trusts, NHS trusts and independent providers of NHS-funded care. Together with the DHSC, NHSI worked to support consistently safe, high quality and compassionate

---

10. By time you read this, NHSI will probably have ended up in the rustbox of ex-NHS organisations. That's what is frustrating about writing a book like this. It's a bit like an 'update on football'.

care (within financially sustainable systems). It was set up on 1 April 2016 following the merging of several organisations including Monitor, NHS Trust Development Authority, and the National Patient Safety Agency.

In April 2018, regional NHSI and NHSE teams combined to create an integrated leadership structure, with 7 regional teams, aiming to enhance local collaboration and efficiency. This merger is nearly complete. Since 1 April 2019, NHSI and NHSE have worked as one organisation, known as NHSE, although they remain legally distinct under the HSC Act 2012.

Care Quality Commission (CQC)
The CQC was established in 2009 to independently register, monitor, inspect and regulate HSC providers including hospitals, care homes, GP surgeries, dental practices and other HSC services in England. All HSC providers are legally required to register with the CQC, who ensure services meet fundamental standards of quality and safety. CQC establishes these standards and publishes performance ratings on a four-point scale: outstanding, good, requires improvement and inadequate. Where standards of care are not met, CQC issues warnings or penalty notices, restrict services, suspends registration or prosecutes the provider.

General Medical Council (GMC)
The Medical Act 1858 established the GMC as the independent regulator of doctors in the UK with the remit:
1. To protect, promote and maintain the health, safety and well-being of the public
2. To protect and promote public confidence in the medical profession
3. To protect and maintain proper professional standards and conduct for members of the medical profession.

These are accomplished by:
- **Medical Register.** It performs identity and qualification checks before a doctor is allowed to the register and practice
- **Standards for Doctors.** It sets the professional values, knowledge, skills and behaviours required
- **Medical Education and Training**. It sets standards for undergraduate and postgraduate medical education
- **Revalidation.** It maintains and improves standards by ensuring doctors have an annual appraisal and undergo revalidation every five years
- **Concerns.** It investigates, addresses and acts on concerns raised about doctors and can issue a warning, restrict practice, enforce retraining or supervision, or erase a doctor from the medical register.

Nursing and Midwifery Council (NMC) and other Councils
The NMC is the independent regulatory body for nurses, midwives and nursing associates. The NMC protects the public by setting standards of practice, maintaining a register, monitoring practice and conduct, quality assurance and education; and investigating complaints about misconduct and fitness to practice.

The governing body of the council consists of twelve members: six lay people and six nurses or midwives from the home nations. The governing body sets the strategic direction of the NMC and takes key decisions.

There are other regulatory bodies for other NHS professions. These include the General Dental Council (GDC), Health and Care Professions Council (HCPC: for allied health professionals, e.g. physiotherapists and occupational therapists), and the General Pharmaceutical Council (GPhC).

Training and Development Bodies

The successful delivery of healthcare services by the NHS is entirely reliant on the capabilities, skills and knowledge of its staff and workforce.

Health Education England (HEE)

According to HEE, it is an autonomous national body with a purpose to:

"support the delivery of excellent healthcare and health improvement to the patients and the public of England by ensuring that the workforce has the right numbers, skills, values and behaviours, at the right time and in the right place".

Some of the functions of HEE include:
- **Workforce planning.** It provides national leadership on the planning and development of the healthcare workforce
- **Promotes high quality education and training.** It makes sure it is responsive to the changing needs of patients and local communities
- **Local Education and Training Boards (LETBs).** HEE appoints, oversees and supports LETBs
- **Allocates NHS education and training funds.** It ensures transparency, fairness and efficiency in investment across England
- **Trained Staff Supply.** HEE makes sure there is an adequate number of professionally qualified staff to run the NHS
- **Innovation.** It assists the spread of innovation across the NHS.

HEE is allocated an annual budget of about £4.5 billion, 70% of which is spent on undergraduate and postgraduate medical and dental education. The budget is distributed to LETBs. The progress of HEE is monitored by the DHSC using the Education Outcomes Framework (EOF).

Local Education and Training Boards (LETBs)

The 13 LETBs (or 'Deaneries') are subcommittees of HEE and are responsible for the training and education of NHS staff within their area. Unfortunately, for historical reasons, these are not the same as the seven NHSE regions[11]. Their function is to bring together healthcare providers in each locality to improve training and education quality.

---

11. Or the 10 Clinical Senates, 4 PHE regions, 14 Ambulance Trusts .. starting to get it?!

The roles of the governing bodies of LETBs include:
- Identify and agree the local needs for education and training
- Plan and commission high quality education and training locally
- Support national workforce priorities set by HEE.

Academy of Royal Colleges and Professional Bodies

The Academy of Medical Royal Colleges (the Academy) is a coordinating body for the UK and Ireland's 23 medical Royal Colleges and Faculties. It ensures safe and proper care by setting standards for medical education, training and monitoring. Many colleges set professional exams for doctors to progress after initial qualification.

Many medical specialties have national professional bodies that are not Royal Colleges or Faculties. These include the British Thoracic Society, British Cardiovascular Society, British Society of Gastroenterology, Renal Association and the Society for Acute Medicine.

Universities

As well as training future healthcare professionals, universities work with the NHS to develop new skills and treatments. This is often the role of *clinical academics*, who work both at an NHS Trust and its affiliated university.

Data and Evidence Gathering
National Institute for Health and Care Excellence (NICE)

NICE was set up initially as the National Institute for Clinical Excellence in April 1999, and on 1 April 2005 joined with the Health Development Agency to become the National Institute for Health and Clinical Excellence. Following the HSC Act 2012, NICE was renamed the National Institute for Health and Care Excellence.

NICE was initially set up to reduce geographical variations in the availability and quality of NHS treatments and care, the 'Postcode Lottery'. However over the years, its role has evolved to provide guidance and thereby improve outcomes for people using HSC services. It has also acquired an international reputation for the development of clinical guidelines. Its three main responsibilities are:

- **Evidence-based Guidelines and Advice.** NICE uses the best available evidence to help develop recommendations that guide public health and HSC including:
  - Clinical Guidelines - provide recommendations about the management and treatment of specific medical conditions
  - Medical Technology - provides recommendations about new medical technologies involved in detecting, monitoring or treating medical conditions
  - Public Health - provides recommendations to prevent disease as well as promote and maintain good health
  - Social Care - provides independent recommendations on the effectiveness and cost-effectiveness of social care interventions and services

- **Standards.** NICE creates legally binding quality standards and performance metrics
- **Information.** NICE provides a range of information for commissioners, clinicians and managers in HSC.

Dr Foster Intelligence
This formed in 2006 to monitor the performance of the NHS and provide computerised healthcare information for the UK public. It also sends alerts to hospitals if it 'sees' an increase in mortality or morbidity.

Medicines Regulation
Cancer Drug Fund (CDF)
The CDF was formed in 2010 initially as a temporary solution to help patients gain access to cancer drugs not routinely funded by the NHS in England but the process quickly became financially unsustainable, and a review of the CDF was carried out.

In the new (2016) model, the CDF functions as a transitional fund, paying for new drugs in advance of a NICE full assessment. During this assessment period, NHSE and NICE work in partnership with pharmaceutical companies to collect additional data concerning the effectiveness of new cancer treatments. Thus, the primary aims of the new CDF are to:
- Provide patients with faster access to the most promising new cancer treatments
- Help ensure value for money
- Offer pharmaceutical companies a fast-track route to NHS funding.

Clinicians can apply on behalf of patients using the NHSE Individual Funding Request (IFR) system. If a drug is given conditional approval, it will move into the CDF for a period of up to two years, while being appraised by NICE.

Medicines and Healthcare products Regulatory Agency (MHRA)
The MHRA is an executive agency of the DHSC. Its main responsibilities are:
- Ensuring medicines, medical devices and blood components for transfusion, meet applicable standards of safety, quality and efficacy
- Ensuring the supply chain for medicines, medical devices and blood components is safe and secure.

Information Technology (IT)

NHS Digital
NHS Digital functions to provide information, data and IT systems for the NHS in England. The duties of NHS digital are:
- Collecting, analysing and publishing health and care data
- Make submitting data as easy as possible for health and care staff
- Providing national technology for health and care services
- Providing information standards

- Improving the quality of health and care information and data
- Publishing national indicators for health and care, to measure quality of care and progress against policy initiatives
- Giving advice and support to health and care organisations on information and cyber security.

NHS digital works closely with NHSE, NHSX, National Information Board, and all parts of the NHS and social care in England.

NHSX
NHSX is a unit with responsibility for setting national policy and developing best practice for NHS technology, digital and data (including data sharing and transparency). It was established in April 2019 to bring together information technology teams from the DHSC, NHSE and NHS Improvement. NHSX works closely with the Government Digital Service and other relevant government agencies.

One of the functions of the organisation is to manage the sharing of NHS patient data with industry. In March 2020, NHSX commissioned a contact tracking app to monitor the spread of C19. The 'X' in NHSX stands for 'user eXperience'.

Healthcare Service Delivery
Primary Care
Primary care services provide the first point of contact in the healthcare system for patients. They primarily see non-urgent cases, and services include GPs, dentists, optometry services and community pharmacies. Their funding is complicated, being commissioned and funded by CCGs and NHSE regions.

Primary care professionals aim to resolve problems locally, preventing illness, making diagnoses and providing treatment. If conditions require more specialised treatment or investigation, then patients are referred to an alternative healthcare provider, usually secondary care.

Primary Care Networks (PCNs)
PCNs were formally established across England in July 2019 to create fully integrated community-based health services. A PCN is usually 5-10 general practices working closely together with a range of local providers to offer coordinated HSC services for (typically) 30-50,000 patients. How they will work with the new subregional entities STP/ICSs is not yet clear.

Secondary and Tertiary Care
Secondary care refers to services usually based in a hospital, although some are also community based. It includes specialist treatment and support provided for patients referred by primary care. This includes both emergency and non-emergency hospital care. Secondary care is commissioned and funded by CCGs.

Tertiary care refers to the larger regional teaching hospitals, whose funding comes partly from the CCGs (70%) and partly from NHS England's regions' specialist commissioning teams (30%).

Mental Health Care
Mental health trusts provide community, inpatient and social services for a wide range of psychiatric and psychological illnesses and are commissioned and funded by CCGs. Mental health services can also be provided by other NHS organisations, the voluntary sector and the private sector.

Community Health Services
Community health services deliver a wide range of services across multiple settings – including people's homes, community clinics, community centres and schools. Community services often support individuals with multiple, complex health needs. They provide a wide range of services including adult community nursing, health visitors, school nursing, community specialist services, therapy services, preventative services (e.g. smoking cessation clinics), sexual health clinics, 'hospital at home', NHS walk-in centres and home-based rehabilitation. Adult community health services are commissioned by CCGs, whilst local authorities commission children's community services.

The funding of social care is complicated and disjointed, coming from a variety of sources, including CCGs and local authorities, as well as individuals. This complexity is part of the reason it is hard to get frail elderly patients home from hospital.

Armed Forces Healthcare
The armed forces include current serving personnel and veterans and their families. Although there is an overlap in the health needs of the armed forces and general population, sometimes significant differences can arise; including health conditions such as depression and post-traumatic stress disorder, which can arise because of things people experience in the services.

Healthcare for veterans and families of service personnel remains the responsibility of the DHSC. In areas where there are large numbers of veterans, specific commissioning of relevant services is required with some service provision led by charities such as 'Help for Heroes' and the Royal British Legion. For serving personnel, healthcare is delivered by the Ministry of Defence (MOD), combined with the NHS, charities and other welfare organisations.

Primary care is delivered by the MOD through the Defence Medical Services (DMS) which functions to promote, protect and restore the health of the UK armed forces so they are medically fit to serve. The DMS provides a wide range of services including primary care, dental care, rehabilitation, occupational medicine, community mental healthcare and specialist medical care. It caters for around 135,360 UK armed forces personnel and is staffed by around 12,100 service and 2,500 civilian personnel.

Secondary care is provided within the NHS by a mixture of military consultants and nurses working within NHS facilities and by NHS staff, e.g. at Queen Alexandra Hospital in Portsmouth, Derriford Hospital in Plymouth, and Queen Elizabeth Hospital in Birmingham.

NHSE Health and Justice (NHSE HJ) - Prisons, etc.

NHSE HJ is responsible for commissioning healthcare in prisons, secure facilities for children and young people, police and court 'Liaison and Diversion (L&D)' services, and immigration removal centres as well as cases of sexual abuse/assault. NHSE HJ teams aim to provide an equal level of service to that offered to the rest of the population.

Prisoners get poor, disjointed healthcare, partly as they are often moved around the country, and partly as it is difficult undertaking investigations or following them up. This is because prison authorities are reluctant to give prisoners planned appointments, which tell the prisoner where they will be and when, as they fear they will abscond.

NHSE HJ tries to establish links with CCGs and local authorities, to support the delivery of care within secure settings, and continuity of care as individuals move about. HJ services are commissioned via 10 HJ teams across 4 regions[12] (North, Midlands, London and South). There are separate health and justice systems for Scotland, Wales and Northern Ireland.

Important Individuals

As well as organisations, there are several important individuals in the NHS. Some of whom became household names during the C19 pandemic.

Secretary of State for Health and Social Care

The Secretary of State for Health, also known as the 'Health Secretary', has the overall responsibility for the work of the DHSC. The Health Secretary has a wide range of duties, including having overall financial control, and oversight of NHS delivery and performance and social care policy in the UK.

Chairman of Health and Social Care Committee

This is a cross-party committee responsible for scrutiny of the DHSC and its associated public bodies.

Chief Medical Officer (CMO)

The CMO is the UK government's principle medical adviser, and professional lead for all doctors employed in England in public health, the Civil Service and the military. There are CMOs for Scotland, Wales, and Northern Ireland. Each CMO is assisted by one or more Deputy Chief Medical Officers.

Chief Nursing Officer (CNO)

The CNO is the professional lead for nurses and midwives in England. Their overarching role is to oversee improvements in patient safety and experience.

Chief Professional Officers

The Chief Professional Officers are the government's heads of profession. They work in NHS England and report to the National Medical Director. These include the Chief

---

12. And another disconnected silo.

Scientific Officer, Chief Dental Officer, Chief Pharmaceutical Officer and Chief Allied Health Professions Officer.

NHSE Chief Executive (CEO)
The CEO of NHSE is accountable to Parliament for NHSE's £130+ billion of annual funding.

NHSE National Medical Director
The National Medical Director for NHSE is the professional lead for all doctors in England with the exception of those employed in public health, the Civil Service or the military. The Medical Director is responsible for clinical policy and strategy, enhancing clinical leadership and promoting innovation.

Healthcare in the Three Nations
Healthcare in Scotland
The Scottish Government Directorate for HSC has responsibility for health policy, the administration of NHS Scotland, community care and some responsibility for social work. The directorate is headed by the Director General for HSC, who is the CEO for NHS Scotland. The directorate sets national objectives and priorities for the NHS, monitors performance and supports boards to ensure achievement of key objectives. NHS Scotland employs 160,000 staff.

Regional NHS Boards
The 14 regional NHS boards in Scotland are responsible for planning, commissioning and delivery of frontline healthcare services, and for health protection and improvement. NHS Boards are accountable to Scottish government ministers (who are, in turn, accountable to the Scottish parliament).

Special Health Boards (SHBs)
The 7 Scottish SHBs main role is to support the regional boards by providing a range of important specialist and national services:
- **Public Health Scotland** - responsible for improving and protecting population health and reducing health inequalities
- **NHS Education for Scotland** - responsible for designing, commissioning and quality assuring education and training
- **NHS National Waiting Times Centre** - ensures prompt access to treatment. It receives referrals from across Scotland to reduce waiting times in key elective specialities
- **NHS 24** - an online and telephone-based information and advice service
- **Scottish Ambulance Service**
- **State Hospitals Board for Scotland** - provides high security forensic and psychiatric care
- **NHS National Services Scotland** - supplies a range of essential services including Scottish Healthcare Supplies, The Scottish Blood Transfusion Service and Health Protection Scotland.

Health Improvement Scotland
Health Improvement Scotland provides advice and guidance on effective clinical practice, sets standards for care, reviews and monitors performance - and is an inspection agency.

Healthcare in Wales
NHS Wales delivers healthcare services through Local Health Boards and National NHS Trusts. NHS Wales is accountable to Welsh ministers and the Community Health Councils, which provide a link between patients and the organisations that deliver services.

Local Health Boards (LHBs)
NHS Wales has seven LHBs, which are responsible for planning, securing and delivering healthcare services. The LHBs aim to integrate specialist, secondary, community and primary care and health improvements.

NHS National Trusts
There are three NHS Trusts in Wales, the Welsh Ambulance Service NHS Trust, Velindre NHS Trust (provides specialist services in cancer and blood services) and Public Health Wales.

Community Health Councils (CHCs)
There are seven CHCs, which give members of the public an independent voice in their local NHS.

Healthcare in Northern Ireland
The Northern Ireland Department of Health has overall responsibility for HSC services provided via the integrated services of Health and Social Care (Northern Ireland).

Health and Social Care Board (HSCB)
The HSCB holds overall responsibility for commissioning services, managing resources and performance improvement. They discharge their responsibilities through five local commissioning groups.

Local Commissioning Group (LCGs)
The LCGs are aligned to the boundaries of five HSC trusts and are responsible for the commissioning of HSC.

Health and Social Care Trusts (HSCTs)
HSCTs have regional responsibility for providing integrated HSC.

Public Health Agency (PHA)
The PHA is the major organisation responsible for health protection and HSC improvement, in Northern Ireland.

Other Organisations
NHS Charities
Even though the majority of NHS funding is through general taxation, many members of the public like to contribute to it through the many NHS official charities. Charities support the NHS in many ways, including providing support and equipment directly to patients and their families, and funding medical research, training and education. 'NHS Charities Together', based in Warwick, represents and supports over 230 of the NHS's official charities. Captain Sir Tom Moore brought this charity to the attention of the public during the C19 pandemic.

Think Tanks
The King's Fund is a health charity that shapes Health and Social Care policy. It is primarily a research charity, whose aim is to:

"achieve extraordinary improvements in health by supporting the brightest minds".

In addition to funding biomedical research, it supports the public understanding of science, e.g. using exhibitions. The Nuffield Trust aims to improve the quality of healthcare in the UK by providing evidence-based research and policy analysis and informing and generating debate.

Royal Society of Medicine (RSM)
This independent and apolitical provider of postgraduate medical education promotes an exchange of information and ideas on the science, practice and organisation of medicine.

Unions
There are about 15 healthcare trade unions in the UK. These include the British Medical Association, Hospital Consultants and Specialists Association, British Dental Association, Royal College of Nursing, and Unison (stylised as UNISON), the largest trade union in the UK with almost 1.4 million members.
  We told you it was complicated!

Further reading
The home page of Healthwatch.

https://www.healthwatch.co.uk/what-we-do

NHS Scotland's homepage.

https://www.scot.nhs.uk/about-nhs-scotland/

NHS Wales's homepage.

http://www.wales.nhs.uk/nhswalesaboutus/structure

Health and Social Care Northern Ireland's homepage.

http://online.hscni.net/home/hsc-structure/

Chapter 6

Specialists and Specialised Commissioning

"You get an ology, you're a scientist!" Maureen Lipman (British Telecom advert, 1987).

This chapter is about people that want an 'ology', i.e. want to specialise, and how the NHS organises and funds Specialised Services.

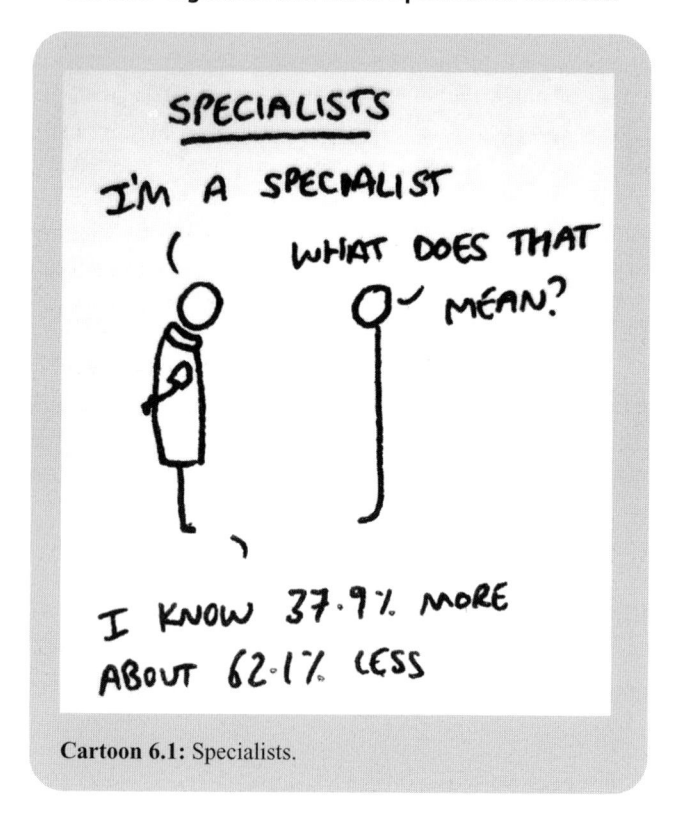

SPECIALISTS

I'M A SPECIALIST

WHAT DOES THAT MEAN?

I KNOW 37.9% MORE ABOUT 62.1% LESS

Cartoon 6.1: Specialists.

Introduction

The following terms *specialist*, *speciality*, *sub-speciality*, *specialised services* and *specialised commissioning* are confusing given they are not interchangeable and require explanation. An initial broad distinction can be made between 'specialist' and 'specialised'. A 'specialist' refers to the level of expertise delivered by a doctor who has undergone specific training. 'Specialised' refers to a form of commissioning used by the NHS to purchase specialised services[13].

What is a Specialist?

Our modern understanding of medical specialisation and specialists began in 19th Century Paris, where an ever-increasing number of doctors pursued specific areas of medicine and declared themselves *specialists* (from the French word 'spécialiste'[14]).

There were numerous reasons for the division of medicine into various 'specialities', including the increasing complexity of medicine and its categorisation into organ-specific pathologies. This creates natural divisions (or specialisms), for institutions and individuals to organise themselves into. We now encounter these *specialisms* daily.

Currently in the UK, a doctor will require several years of clinical practice, training, research, studying and post-graduate exams to become a specialist. There are currently over 60 recognised medical specialities including cardiology, nephrology, anaesthetics, general surgery, ophthalmology - which take between 3-8 years (after the completion of foundation year training) for a doctor to train in.

Speciality training is described in more detail in Chapter 4. During speciality training, a doctor can pursue training in a sub-speciality (a narrower field of the speciality). Most specialities have numerous sub-specialities, e.g. within cardiology: interventional cardiology, electrophysiology, heart failure and congenital heart disease.

On completion of their speciality training, the doctor receives a Certificate of Completion of Specialist Training (CCST) and can apply to be listed on the GMC's Specialist Register and as a result can be appointed as a Consultant.

There are specialist posts in nursing, and other allied health professionals, although the routes to attaining these titles are not so well defined.

Generalists

General Practitioners (GPs) also undertake several years of training and are placed onto the GMC's GP Register[15]. GPs are referred to as 'generalists', rather than specialists, although they have specialised in the field of General Practice. Being a generalist is not an easy option. It is harder to be knowledgeable about 15 branches of medicine, rather than about one.

Some branches of hospital medicine, including Pathology, Geriatrics, Radiology, Acute and Emergency Medicine, require generalist skills too.

---

13. And yes, this chapter is either more or less interesting than it sounds. Warning: it is acronym-positive!
14. Most medical words go back to the Ancient Greek (and before). So this is an unusually 'new' one. We digress. Again.
15. The Specialist Register and Generalist Register are a benchmark that must be achieved for employers to employ a doctor as an independent and autonomous practitioner.

What is Specialised Commissioning and a Specialised Service?
Background to Specialised Commissioning
The commissioning of specialised services is conducted at a national (and regional) level by NHSE who determine policy and strategy objectives, manage existing specialised services, and manage the process to consider potential specialised services for commissioning.

Seven regional Specialised Commissioning teams (one per region) exist to deliver the strategy developed by the national team, and to secure best value provision of services in line with national standards. The Regions have contracts for specialised services from providers (mainly hospitals); and for this, they use what is called the 'NHS Standard Contract'. Regional teams also provide operational support for the delivery of these services.

The 'NHS Standard Contract' is mandated by NHSE for all healthcare services. There are general conditions within it which set out nationally based terms, although some are set locally. This approach is not used for primary care.

Prior to discussing the definition of a specialised service, it is important to understand the NHSE definition of commissioning:

> "at its simplest, commissioning is the process of planning, agreeing and monitoring services"

> "Commissioning is not one action but many, ranging from the health-needs assessment for a population, through the clinically-based design of patient pathways, to service specification and contract negotiation and procurement, with continuous quality assessment".

Commissioning is (well, should be) therefore a multi-faceted continuous process that assesses the needs of a population; including planning and procurement of services, and monitoring of the quality of the service. Although the cynic would say that often commissioning 'follows' a service developed to meet a local need, e.g. if enough people in a region of the UK have heart failure that requires a heart operation, a cardio-thoracic surgery service develops, and someone has to pay for it.

Where does Specialised Commissioning take place?
The National Specialised Commissioning team, statutorily called the 'NHS Commissioning Board', negotiate contracts (usually yearly) directly with providers. For most acute specialised services, these negotiations are with NHS Trusts (due to the significant requirement to co-locate services). For Mental Health and Learning Disability Services, the market is more mixed with NHS and Independent providers.

It is more complicated than it looks, as the rules are different between England and the three nations. For simplicity, we will focus on the NHS in England, which is overseen by the DHSC and NHSE.

Cost of Specialised Services

NHSE publish a Manual for Prescribed Specialised Services, which states the services funded by specialist commissioning. The 2018/2019 version describes 149 services. The budget in 20/21 was £20.5 billion (c. 17% of the NHS budget) and is projected to grow to £25 billion by 2025. The growth in high-cost drugs is a material contributor to the cost; because NHSE commissions a large proportion of high-cost drugs for cancer therapies, metabolic diseases and immunosuppressants.

Specialised Services are often provided when other options have failed. However, in terms of outcomes, money spent in general practice and mental health (for example), delivers a higher level of benefit pound-for-pound than money spent on specialised services. But, disinvestment from specialised services is difficult, largely due to enhanced patient knowledge and expectation. For example, to dialyse one patient for one year costs around £30,000 and is a recurring cost. And this is money which could be used to support disease prevention initiatives, e.g. reducing obesity, smoking, etc. But stopping dialysis is not really an option.

In its broadest sense, specialised services will have at least one of the following features:
- They treat rare conditions, which only a few doctors have expertise in
- They are expensive
- The infrastructure required to deliver the services requires planning on a geographical scale bigger than a local commissioner (i.e. CCG)
- Because of a large degree of sub-specialism for the clinical teams, services are centralised into fewer providers.

The services include complex medical and surgical conditions (e.g. cardiac and neurosurgery), radiotherapy, surgery and chemotherapy for cancers, treatment of genetic disorders, transplantation, kidney dialysis and a range of cutting-edge drugs, therapies and procedures. Within mental health, Specialised Mental Health Services (e.g. Secure Services) form most non-acute costs, in addition to Learning Disability residential care.

Most specialised services are co-located mainly within teaching hospitals which provide a variety of local, more generalised services. But sometimes they exist as 'standalone' (usually single disease) institutions, like Moorfields Eye Hospital.

Definition of a 'Specialised Service'

A service provided by a group of specialists does not become a 'specialised service' by its own volition. The use of the term 'specialised service' has changed, and its current definition originates in 1996, with further development in the HSC Act 2012. Four statutory factors determine whether a service is designated as specialised:
- The number of patients requiring the service or facility
- The cost of providing the service or the facility
- The number of persons able to provide the service or the facility
- The financial implications for CCGs if they were expected to provide the service or facility.

For a service to become specialised (in a commissioning sense), it must be defined as a 'specialised service' by NHSE. The Prescribed Specialised Services Advisory Group (PSSAG) make recommendations to government about new specialised services.

Examples

Although a specialist practices a certain speciality, this does not necessarily mean that they are delivering a specialised service. For example, a 'normal' cardiology consultant in a DGH is considered a specialist, but the income funding their care is not counted as 'specialised'. So their funding comes from the local CCG. Whereas a cardiothoracic surgeon, who works in a larger teaching hospital, who has patients referred to them by the previously described cardiologist, is considered 'specialised' and is therefore funded via a Regional NHSE Specialised Commissioning Team.

Coordination of Specialised Services

Identifying Specialised Services - Programmes of Care (PoC)

Services are identified as 'specialised' by The Manual for Prescribed Services, which is supplemented by the 'Prescribed Specialised Services Identification Rules'. This creates huge advantages for the specialists and patients in that area, as funding is nationally consistent. Thus, once a service 'gets on the list', it is difficult to remove. This can only be removed by amendment to HSC Act 2012 – as was the case for Bariatric Surgery in 2015.

The management and commissioning of specialised services are arranged into themes that are overseen by six National Programmes of Care (NPoCs):
- Mental Health and Learning Disabilities
- Acute (consists of five separate NPoCs)
    - Trauma
    - Cancer
    - Women and Childrens'
    - Internal Medicine
    - Blood and Infection.

The role of each NPoC is to prioritise and coordinate its services and develop strategy and policy objectives to advise NHSE. Each NPoC receives further support from several Clinical Reference Groups (CRGs) which provide speciality-specific clinical advice and leadership, and contribute to the development of commissioning 'products'. The 'products of commissioning' are sets of rules used by commissioning teams to contract services. They include:
- **Service Specifications.** These define the standards of care an organisation funded by NHSE must display to provide a specialised service
- **Clinical commissioning policies and statements.** These display the inclusion and exclusion criteria that determine access to a service
- **Quality dashboards.** These are standards for judging the efficacy of a specialised service, comparing each unit to national standards and each other.

Each NPoC and CRG consists of a board formed of clinicians (mainly doctors in that specialty), patient and public voice representatives (PPVs), public health doctors, commissioners and managers. They have specific terms of reference and a finite term in office. Most recently, leaders were appointed for a 2-year period after a process which invited expressions of interest[16].

Quality Assessment (QA) of Specialised Services
The internal assessment of the quality of specialised services is done through the Quality Surveillance Information System (or 'QSIS portal'). This involves self-assessments, and a quality dashboard. The data produced is available on-line, but it is hard to find and interpret.

Introduction of New Treatments
New drugs, devices and technologies can improve the treatment of already treatable or treat previously untreatable conditions - but are often expensive. This means difficult decisions need to be made by the NHS as to whether to commission new treatments locally, nationally or not at all. Processes exist to evaluate the clinical and cost effectiveness of these treatments within NICE and NHSE.

NICE Appraisal Process
NICE conducts technology appraisals (TAs) and Highly Specialised Treatment (HST) evaluations and provides recommendations to the NHS on whether a treatment should be funded. NHSE is legally obliged to fund drugs and technologies recommended by TAs and HSTs.

NHSE has its own commissioning process for new treatments, technologies and devices not considered by the TA or HST process. This process utilises Clinical Priority Advisory Groups (CPAGs), which are advisory boards consisting of clinical, commissioning, public health and financial experts as well as 'patient and public voices' (PPVs). CPAGs make their recommendations to the Specialised Commissioning Oversight Group (SCOG), who review these recommendations against the budget available. SCOG then submits its recommendations to NHSE's Specialised Services Commissioning Committee (SSCC) who make the final decision. Simple.

Their combined expertise is used to provide recommendations to NHSE's Executive Board, on whether new specialised services and treatments should be prioritised for funding.

Further Specialisation - Highly Specialised Services (HSSs)
There is a different, national, system for the funding of HSSs which provide care to a small population (under 500 people per year) via a small number of centres. This is to concentrate, maintain and maximise clinical expertise and experience. Some examples of

---

16. If you are thinking 'is this an unnecessarily complex system designed and run by specialists (doctors) to guarantee funding of their team (and their continued employment)?', you may not be far off the truth. And AS is a specialist!

HSS include paediatric and adult heart transplantation, liver transplantation and treatment of rare genetic conditions.

These are about 65 HSSs, those disease groups where there are five or less providers (e.g. hospitals) treating such patients, e.g. Proton Beam Therapy providers. A small number of services are funded overseas, e.g. patients with severe combined immunodeficiency (SCID) are cared for in Milan.

HSS are commissioned by the Highly Specialised Commissioning Team with support from regional teams. The Rare Diseases Advisory Group (RDAG) provides advice to the CPAG on which HSS should continue to be commissioned or become newly commissioned. RDAG also provides advice to the devolved administrations of Northern Ireland, Scotland and Wales.

Other Advisory Groups
High-Cost Drugs
There is also something called the National Tariff Payment System (NTPS) which generates a list of expensive drugs that can be prescribed for the whole of the UK. This is not really part of specialised commissioning but many of these drugs can only be prescribed by specialised service teams.

Other Groupings
'Natural' Healthcare Groupings
In England there are about 10 'natural' healthcare groupings. These are partly geographical and partly historical. For example, there is a 'north of the East Midlands natural group, based around Sheffield' (this exists for deaneries and lines of referral) that is not recognised by NHSE or Specialised Commissioning. In this area, for example, patients in north Nottinghamshire may be referred by their GP to Sheffield (in NHSE Northeast and Yorkshire) for their specialist care, rather than Nottingham (in NHSE Midlands). So a Sheffield hospital may have to obtain finance for a patient's 'general care' from a Nottinghamshire CCG (in NHSE Midlands) and 'Specialised Services' from NHSE NE and Yorkshire.

People that live in 'border areas' between natural health groupings often get less good healthcare and it is your job to spot that and help them. This is partly as they have information on different non-linked computer systems.

Educational Groupings
The specialist commissioning system also has no overlap with the 13 Local Education and Training Boards (LTEBs) 'regions' of HEE. These 'deaneries' train the staff to work in the specialised services. The number 13 is interesting, as the LETBs probably relate to the original 14 Regional Health Boards of the NHS in 1948.

Advantages and Disadvantages of Specialised Commissioning
Advantages
- Consistency
- Fairness (reducing the 'postcode lottery')

- Definitions
- Provide a 'larger footprint' to plan a service
- Planning
- Maintaining resources for specialist care
- Pro-democratic.

Disadvantages
- Requires a separate bureaucracy
- Needs separate financial arrangements
- Efficacy of services is difficult to assess
- System works across, and not with:
  - Educational Groups (e.g. deaneries, see below)
  - 'Natural' Healthcare Groupings (see below)
- Investment in larger teaching hospitals becomes a self-fulfilling prophecy
- Over-focus on rare/expensive diseases/treatments (e.g. by supporting trials on newer drugs, devices or procedures), works against common diseases
- Anti-democratic. There is no open debate on the needs of the majority vs the minority.

History of Specialised Commissioning

Some of this section is based on an article written by Nigel Edwards, Chief Executive of the Nuffield Trust, on the history of specialised commissioning[17].

Early History

To some degree, there has always been a level of national coordination of specialised services, although its exact origins remain hazy. It is logical to separate funding for specialised services that have a high price tag; and which could decimate a smaller local healthcare system's budget.

Interestingly, there was evidence of discussion and planning regarding specialised commissioning from the earliest days of the NHS 'Development of Specialist Services' (Picture 6.1). This is amongst the most important (and rare) early planning documents of the NHS. The phrase 'RHB' on it stands for Regional Health Board, 14 of which formed in the new NHS. It was issued in January 1948 before the NHS began. Clearly such institutions felt their care was so important (and expensive) they needed a different financial arrangement.

One of the key statements in the report was:

"Background General Plan. The planning of the specialist services is one of the primary duties of the Regional Hospital Boards, but it is a task which must clearly be carried out in close collaboration with the Teaching Hospitals. Each of the 14 Regional Boards will normally provide a complete range of specialist medical service within its region."

---

17. https://www.nuffieldtrust.org.uk/news-item/specialised-commissioning-lessons-from-history-and-looking-to-the-future

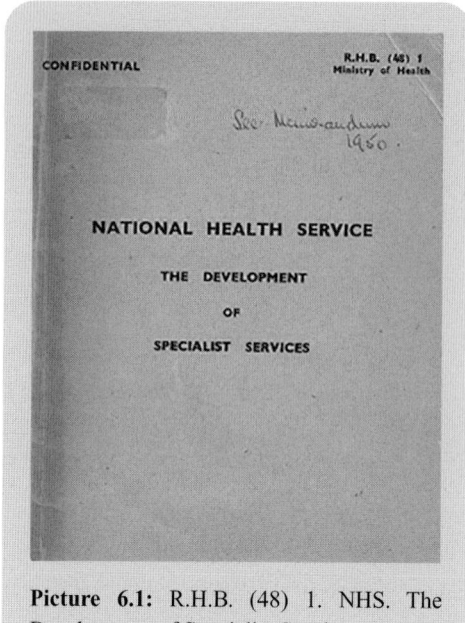

So, it was clear when the NHS formed in 1948, there had already been discussion on the issue. There was also a feeling of responsibility (i.e. it's our job) to provide specialised services, amongst the 36 named teaching hospitals. They accepted (and wanted) co-ordination by the 14 new RHBs, which is largely how specialist care is provided today. In other words, it is carried out in the teaching hospitals, being co-ordinated (and now paid for) by NHSE Regions in the form of their Specialised Commissioning Teams.

The main difference is that there are 7 NHSE regions. There continues to be an assumption not all hospitals within a region will provide specialised services. However - due to a significant increase in scope driven by Lansley's 2012 reforms - in reality some services not typically thought of as 'specialised' (e.g. chemotherapy, HIV, other medical specialties), are provided in almost all hospitals and are *de facto* 'specialised'.

Picture 6.1: R.H.B. (48) 1. NHS. The Development of Specialist Services.

Back to R.H.B. (48) 1. The Ministry of Health (i.e. forerunner of 'DH' and current DHSC) reproduced it in 1950 with minor revisions, including more paragraphs, and in a normal printed format. Some reflected that time had moved on, and the RHBs were up and running. The title was changed to 'The Development of Consultant Services', and it sold for ninepence. Some appendices and maps were added.

1983-1996

"Clearly there had been some form of national level planning of specialised services (not called commissioning) from the early days. But it was not until 1983, that the Supra Regional Services Advisory Group (SRSAG) was established. The definition of what constitutes specialised services has changed over the years - becoming broader or narrower depending on the objectives of policymakers, and the success of different patient, or other lobby, groups in getting their service included." (Nigel Edwards)

Ken Clarke MP (Minister of Health, 1988-90) described the function of the new SRSAG in the House of Commons on 21 January 1983:

"We intend to introduce arrangements by which the financial allocations to certain important services which need to be planned on a national rather than a regional scale will be determined centrally and identified separately from the normal allocations of the health authorities concerned. As part of these arrangements we intend to establish a forum, comprising representatives of health authorities and the medical profession, to advise us on the claims of particular services for supra-regional funding and the level of funding they should receive."

The first four services advised on were: paediatric renal dialysis and transplantation, spinal services, choriocarcinoma and the national poisons information service.

1996-2012

Following the SRSAG, national and regional planning groups slowly developed. The first more formal system started in 1996, when the National Specialised Commissioning Group (NSCG) and ten regionally based Specialised Commissioning Groups (SCGs) were formed. This was probably the first time the phrase 'commissioning' was associated with the process of planning specialised services.

Under this system, the SCGs would collaborate with their counterpart regional Strategic Health Authorities (SHAs) and Primary Care Trusts (PCTs) from 2001 (as they formed) - to commission specialised services according to local needs. The NSCG was responsible for overseeing the regional and national organisation of specialised services.

A sub-committee of the NSCG, called National Commissioning Group (NCG), formed in April 2007. It commissioned a variety of national specialised services. The National Specialised Commissioning Team (NSCT) was responsible for commissioning highly specialised services on behalf of the NCG. The London SHA hosted national specialised services and coordinated the services for all SHAs in England.

A specialised service was then defined in legislature, as a service covering a population of more than one million. A Specialised Services National Definition Set (SSNDS) existed and described 34 services that were considered as specialised.

Sir David Carter, a surgeon and previous Chief Medical Officer for Scotland, conducted a review of specialised commissioning in 2006. He:

> "recommended PCTs pool their risks and create consortia to do specialist commissioning at regional and national level".

Carter also found that PCTs were very poor at cooperating, which in turn created difficulties; including tertiary centres managing many different inclusion and exclusion criteria, or other aspects of pathway or commissioning policy.

> "Clearly smaller-scale organisations have long struggled with specialised commissioning. The mismatch between needs-based allocation and historic patterns of spending becomes a problem for budgetary control, as local commissioners whose populations had high rates of use of these services had no methods for controlling utilisation". (Nigel Edwards)

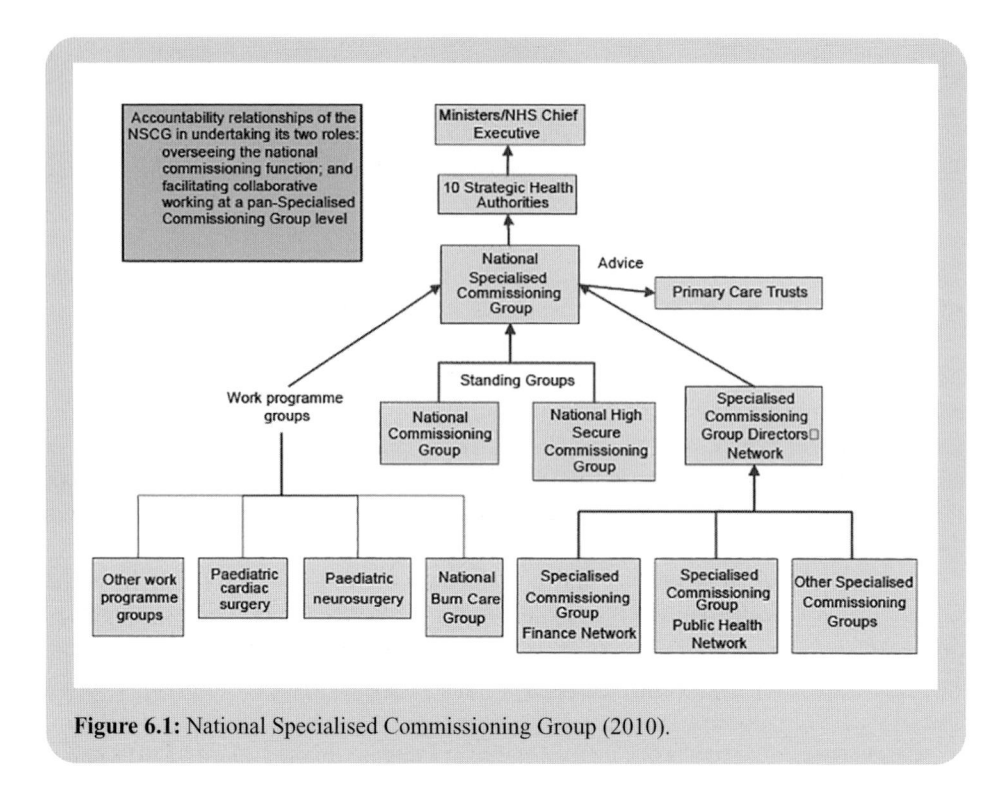

Figure 6.1: National Specialised Commissioning Group (2010).

Carter realised this, as did the Health Select Committee (of the House of Commons) who debated the work of the NSCG in 2010. This discussed why there is an approximate 'right size' for planning specialised services (discussed more later). Figure 6.1 above was part of that discussion.

2012 and Onwards
In 2012, the report: 'Securing Equity and Excellence in Commissioning Specialised Services' was published by NHSE describing the operating model. This was enacted in 2013 through the Health and Social Care Act 2012. As stated earlier, the concept of (and name) 'specialised commissioning' had been established before the 2012 Act, which incorporated much of the report. It was clear at this point there would have to be a system that the local level of administration (CCGs) would not be involved with. It would have its own administration, funding lines, and quality assessment. This is largely how it is organised today. In other words, the 4 NHS regions (later 7) formed in this re-organisation, developed specialised commissioning teams, which still exist.

The 'Report of the Specialised Services Commission' was published in 2016 by Lord Warner. One recommendation it made was that:

> "The management of many specialised services should be delegated to regional and local (CCG) levels, with national management retained primarily for complex specialised services and highly specialised services (NHSE/Ministers)".

This was largely the status quo. It also recommended:

> "Comprehensive cost and key outcomes performance data must form an integral part of these changes, for example by recognising the importance of databases in monitoring and driving performance (NHSE/NHSI)".

In other words, it tended to agree with the view above that monitoring needs to improve and become more transparent.

Specialised Services in the Future (and 'right size' for specialised commissioning)

How specialised services will be co-ordinated in the future is unclear. The debate on the 'right size' for specialised commissioning will continue. The 14 Regions of the 1948 NHS, from where it all started, was (and may still be) 'about right'. They would now serve about four million people each.

The new(ish) seven NHSE Regions may continue to do it. But they are probably too large, serving 14 million-ish each. The 42 subregional Integrated Care Systems (ICSs) (serving over 1 million), as they form, may take over. But they are probably too small. Also ICSs and CCGs (serving about 200,000) are currently light on the infrastructure required to commission specialised services.

Or NHSE regions could work with ICSs to pool commissioning expertise. For example, ICS staff could contribute to a wider pool of knowledge and develop individual areas of specialised commissioning interest on behalf of the region. In other words, there may be a 'lead ICS' for a region, which is responsible for a named specialised service (e.g. cardio-thoracic surgery or renal service). Whatever happens, the need for specialised services will continue and, likely, increase.

Further reading

The Nuffield Trust hosting of the R.H.B. (48) 1. NHS. The Development of Specialist Services.

https://www.nuffieldtrust.org.uk/files/2019-11/nhs-history-book/48-57/rhb481.html

The Warner Report on specialised services commissioning.

http://www.shca.info/perch/resources/specialised-services-commission-report-final-2.pdf

Chapter 7

Mental Health

"We take care of our dental health. We don't take care of our mental health ... I think the solution to making this world better is if we would just be healthy mentally." Howie Mandel (Canadian writer and comedian).

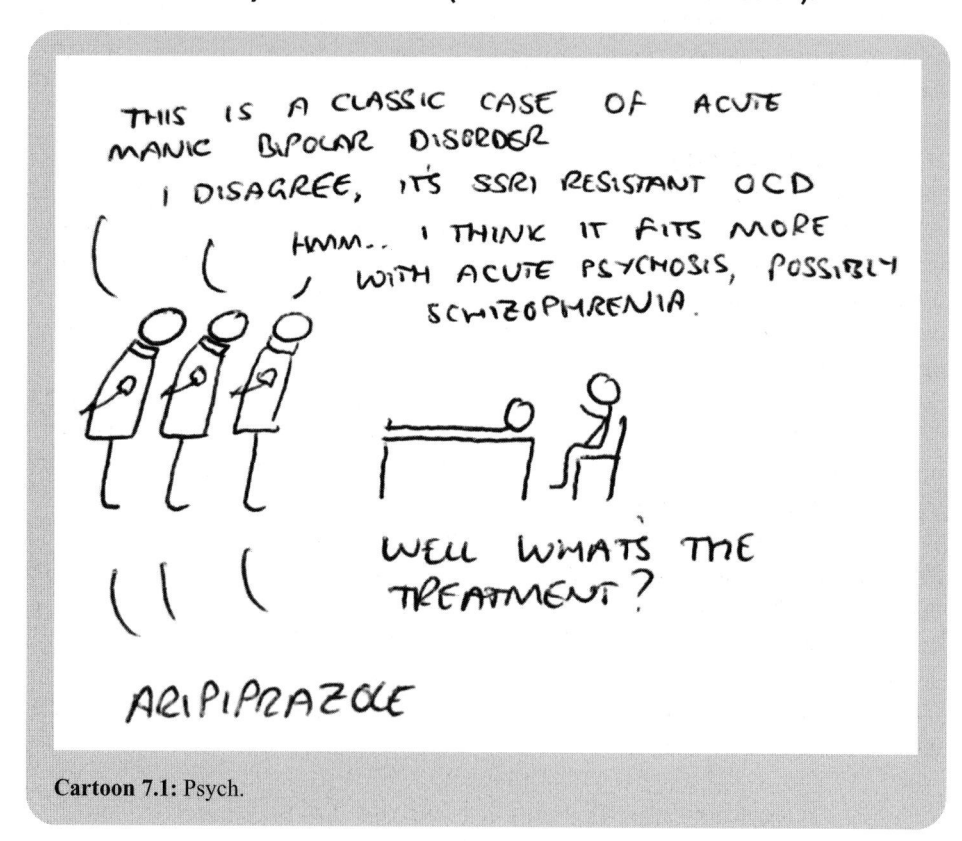

Cartoon 7.1: Psych.

What is Mental Health?

Mental health is defined, by the WHO, as a

> "state of well-being in which every individual realises his or her own potential, can cope with the normal stresses of life, can work productively and fruitfully, and is able to make a contribution to her or his community".

Elements of the mind such as emotions, cognitive function, behaviour, and social well-being are key to the evaluation of the mental state. Despite affecting one in four people annually, there is a social stigma surrounding mental health problems, with people with mental health issues often seen in a negative light and regarded as dangerous.

Epidemiology

The prevalence of mental illnesses is very high. It is the largest single cause of disability, although waiting for treatment can take up to a year. One in six of those affected by mental health issues are working-age adults experiencing issues such as depression, generalised anxiety, and panic disorders. Around 602,000 cases of mental health illness were linked to work-related stress, depression, and anxiety in 2018/2019. In 2019, men aged 40-49 years old had the highest suicide rate within the UK. For 16-19 year olds in an intimate relationship, almost 25% have experienced physical abuse impacting their mental health.

History of Psychiatry

In early Medieval times, there was no differentiation between medicine, magic, and religion. It was thought, for example, that by 'letting out the evil spirit', one could cure madness. In the early 15th through to the 17th century, those suffering mental illness were often thought of as witches. During the 19th century, Kraepelin and Alzheimer discovered methods to identify neurological diseases, and developed ideas for a framework for psychiatric conditions (based on presentations and outcomes).

Mental health services existed before the NHS, with their work mandated by the 1890 Lunacy Act. This followed the act of the same name of 1845 which had established people who suffered mental illness as patients. The first UK Mental Health Act was passed in 1959 (amended in 1983 and 2007).

A National Service Framework was developed for adult mental health in 1999, and for children and young people in 2004. For older adults, an integrated framework was developed in 2006; when it was noted that significantly more money was being spent on physical health, particularly in children and elderly care. This in part spurred on the development of the Improving Access to Psychological Therapies (IAPT) programme in 2006; increasing access to primary care psychological therapies - especially for mild to moderate mental health illness.

Primary, Secondary and Tertiary Mental Health Services

Mental health services can be accessed through different tiers of the NHS. Secondary care services, based in hospitals and the community, are seen as specialist and receive referrals from primary care. Tertiary care includes highly specialised mental health services, such as forensic mental health. Acute Trusts, via Emergency Departments and Walk-in centres, are also able to provide mental health services. Mental health liaison services (e.g. for patients experiencing a mental health crisis) can be based in psychiatric hospitals but also work in acute hospitals.

Primary Care Mental Health Service

It is estimated nearly 3 million adults are newly diagnosed with depression per year, making it the commonest chronic condition in the UK. There has been a steady increase in the use of antidepressants. In 2017-2018, nearly 7,300,000 adults were prescribed antidepressants in England. 500,000 people are diagnosed annually with severe mental illnesses (SMI), e.g. with conditions such as schizophrenia and bipolar disorder. Primary care has an important role in identifying signs of SMI; and ensuring people are guided to, and supported through, an individualised treatment programme.

Improving Access to Psychological Therapy (IAPT)
The NHS's IAPT programme started in 2008 providing psychological therapy at a primary care level. IAPT practitioners are trained psychological therapists who help people cope with life, work and mental illnesses. Notably people with chronic physical illness are at high risk of developing depression and anxiety. IAPT is usually based on cognitive behavioural therapy (CBT) but can also offer supportive counselling. IAPT interventions are recommended by the National Institute of Health and Care Excellence (NICE).

The purpose of IAPT is to help individuals adapt and cope with long and short-term conditions; as well as reducing inequality, and improving outcomes in particular population groups. IAPT aims to reach 1.9 million adults annually.

Digital Enabled Therapy (DET)
DETs are therapies accessed online and via mobile applications (which makes DETs highly accessible). They can be used to reinforce self-study based programmes or can be supported by trained therapists. Most DET programmes focus on common disorders such as depression and anxiety. There are also a limited number of specialised digital programmes for more complex mental health problems.

'Velibra' is designed to help people suffering from generalised social anxiety and panic disorders. It has proven to be more effective when integrated into a general support plan. Such programmes aim to support more independent people, allowing mental health practitioners to help more dependent ones.

There are multiple online programmes available for adults with depression. *'Space'*, *'Deprexis'*, and *'Minddistrict'* are NICE recommended and based on CBT; whilst *'Regul8'* is an online CBT-based programme designed to help those with Irritable Bowel Syndrome.

Secondary Care Mental Health Service

Secondary care mental health services care for patients whose conditions are complex. They are provided by a combination of liaison psychiatry (working in acute hospitals), inpatient psychiatry, and community care.

Liaison Psychiatry
Liaison psychiatry focuses on the link between the patient's physical and mental health and is commonly found in acute hospitals. Patients may present with a mental health crisis such as overdose, self-harm or a relapse of an SMI (like psychosis). For example,

individuals who come into the ED with an overdose or serious self-harm, are initially managed by 'front-end' teams and stabilised; and then transferred to the liaison psychiatry team. Early intervention can decrease hospital stays and is therefore cost-effective.

Community-based Care
Community Mental Health Teams (CMHTs) and Crisis Resolution and Home Treatment teams (CRHTs) are part of secondary care, and have transformed and modernised mental health care.

Psychiatric Inpatient Care
About 35% of patients admitted to psychiatric wards are detained under a 'section' of the Mental Health Act 1983, when they are acutely unwell. Services provided to inpatients include:
- Intensive Short Stay Rehabilitation
- Community Inpatient Services
- Slow Stream Rehabilitation
- Psychiatric Intensive Care Units (PICUs)
- Acute Psychiatry.

On admission, a patient is allocated to a named nurse with whom they will have one-to-one sessions, and they are reviewed on medical ward rounds. Care coordinators (a key worker from their community team) will work closely with inpatients and are also involved in their discharge planning.

As an inpatient, a patient may also receive interventions which include medication, art therapy and life skills training. Discharge planning is commenced soon after a patient is admitted, with options for discharge including discharge-to-home, a rehabilitation unit or supported living environment. Throughout the inpatient stay, the patient is involved in shared decision making regarding their care.

Tertiary Care Mental Health Service
Tertiary services are specialised areas and include:
- Forensic Mental Health Teams
- Children and Adolescent Mental Health Services (CAMHs) Inpatient Services.

Forensic Mental Health Teams
The first forensic mental health hospital in England was Broadmoor Criminal Lunatic Asylum, which opened in 1863. Forensic mental health services care for patients who have a mental illness that poses a risk to others. These services are usually found in secure hospitals, the community and prisons. They work closely with primary care, social care, and the criminal justice system - to reduce re-offending and enable safe discharge.

Mental health services in prisons are like those within any community-based setting and include mental health in-reach teams (MHITs). If compulsory treatment is required, prisoners are transferred to a secure hospital in England and Wales. Most forensic mental health services are provided by the NHS; but in Scotland, the independent sector also contributes.

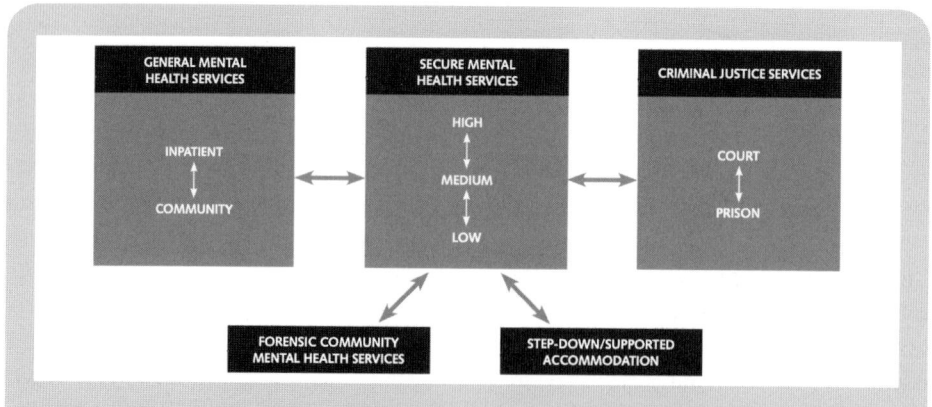

Figure 7.1: Pathways in mental health connecting to the criminal justice system. Taken from: JCPMH -Guidance for commissioners of forensic mental health services.

Inpatient services include 'low', 'medium' and 'high' secure care. Any individual admitted to an inpatient service is detained under the Mental Health Act 1983; and may remain detained for up to two years, with most having been sentenced to detention by the courts.

There are 'Low Secure Units' for adults who have chronic and complex mental health problems that cannot be managed effectively in acute inpatient settings. Referrals are made from PICUs, medium secure services and the criminal justice system.

'Medium Secure Units' treat patients who have SMIs and pose a risk to themselves and others. Transferring from a low to medium security unit may occur due to an increase in the complexity of their needs. Most are referred after court proceedings, or from PICU and other mental health services.

In a 'High Secure Unit', all patients are admitted under the Mental Health Act 1983; and meet the criteria of the NHS Act 2006, having violent and criminal tendencies. 'Long stays' in high secure facilities are defined as being for a minimum of 10 years.

The Bradley Report 2009

The Bradley Report 2009 acknowledged offenders who had both SMIs and less severe mental health disorders can be treated safely in the community by Criminal Justice Mental Health Teams; which help individuals within the justice system to get into contact with their GP or local mental health service. Collaborative working is essential to ensure the individual is supported and managed appropriately.

Children's Inpatient Service

The Children and Adolescent Mental Health Service (CAMHS) provides care in the community, or inpatient setting. But this is only for as long as required (to decrease disruption to the child's life, e.g. education) and as close to home as possible.

The NHS Mental Health Implementation Plan (2019) provided a strategy to reduce the number of children and young people requiring inpatient care. This involves early identification, investigation and management. CAMHS provide a range of services. These include:

- High Dependency Units / PICU
- Eating Disorder Units
- General Adolescent Units
- Specialist Learning Disabilities and Autism Units.

Most units do not admit children under the age of 13 years.

Community Mental Health Care

In England, the NHS Long Term Plan 2019 aims for a more collaborative and seamless service between primary and secondary care, including mental health. CMHTs will work as part of new sub-regional Integrated Care Systems (ICS); allowing for better population-based planning, funding and delivery of local healthcare.

Some of the community services currently provided include:
- Psychological therapy
- Medical assessment and management
- Physical health checks
- Social and fitness groups
- Occupational therapy
- Support with finances, housing, etc.

The following teams may be involved.

Community Mental Health Team (CMHT)
CMHTs are usually accessed via a single point of access (or 'access hubs') which GPs, healthcare or social care professionals, and sometimes patients or their relatives, can refer to them. To prevent delays to those at high risk, questions regarding suicidal thoughts, deliberate self-harm, dependent children and risk to others, are all assessed.

Assertive Outreach Teams (AOT)
This service is often separate from, but sometimes incorporated into, CMHTs. An AOT is a specialised team working with individuals who struggle to engage with mental health services. They may have had several hospital admissions and a history of violence, self-harm or substance abuse. The team provides long-term, intensive support by helping with daily living activities; e.g. support for cleaning their home, taking medication, and access to CBT programmes. AOTs are also able to help in finding education, employment and training opportunities.

Patients with SMIs who get support from AOTs may engage with an Individual Placement and Support (IPS) plan, providing in-work support for both the employee and the employer.

Early Intervention to Psychosis (EIP) Team
EIP teams work with adolescents and adults up to the age of 35 years who experience a first episode, or who are at high risk, of developing a first episode of psychosis. 31.7 per 100,000 people experience their first episode of psychosis each year in the UK.

The more episodes of psychosis a person has, and the longer these are left untreated, the poorer the prognosis. Early intervention teams aim to start treatment quickly (the aim is for within two weeks of referral), provide psychoeducation to patients and their families, and support young people with education, employment and hobbies.

Crisis Resolution and Home Treatment (CRHT) Team
CRHT teams are multidisciplinary and respond to people who require urgent 24 hours and 7 days a week support, e.g. for an episode of psychosis (like schizophrenia), severe self-harm, or a suicide attempt. CRHT teams develop plans to help prevent future crises and administer medication. CRHTs work closely with carers, families and friends; knowing their support will help with a patient's recovery.

CRHTs also provide support to CMHTs when patients require a more intense level of support. One important aim of CRHTs is to provide an alternative to hospital admission. This includes supporting patients who are on leave from the hospital, or who have recently been discharged.

Care Programme Approach (CPA)
The CPA is an enhanced care pathway for people with mental illnesses who may need an extra, or more structured, support plan provided by a care coordinator. Other professionals involved in the patient's care will have copies of their support plan and may be invited to care plan reviews.

Voluntary, Community and Social Enterprises (VCSEs)
Mental health services rely on the important work of VCSEs to support people with mental illness. They cover a wide range of domains including employment, housing and peer support.

Mind is an independent charitable organisation that offers a range of services which include:
- Crisis Service
- Abuse Support
- Addiction services
- Advocacy
- Bereavement
- Housing
- Learning Disability
- LGBTIQ Mental Health
- Counselling and other Talking Therapies
- Peer Support.

Mind also signpost other forms of support and help regarding mental health.

Recovery Academies provide patients, and their carers, with courses and workshops that help the patient's journey towards recovery. They are often run either by (or in conjunction with) local mental health trusts or other services such as Mind. They offer courses and workshops on topics such as:
- Psychological Therapies and Recovery
- Physical Wellbeing
- Spirituality and Recovery
- Creativity and Recovery
- Taking Back Control
- Developing Knowledge and Life Skills
- Addiction
- Identity and Self Esteem.

Age UK is a charity which provides support and services for people over 60 years. They make people aware of what help is available, e.g. information on wellbeing and health and care.

Older Mental Health Services
With increasing life expectancy, there is increasing vulnerability to complex illnesses such as dementia and depression.

Older Adult Mental Health Services provide care in several settings, such as primary care, general hospitals, hospices, and prisons. Such services do not just help with mental health problems but also help promote wellbeing and health generally. Depression, suicidal feelings and substance abuse are very common in older people, all of which are managed by older adult mental health services.

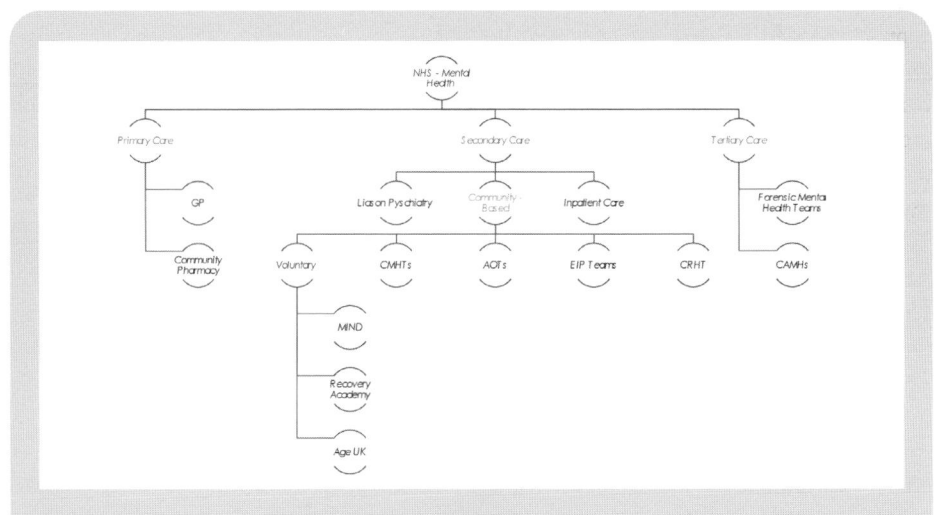

Figure 7.2: Summary of England's Mental Health Services.

Summary of Structure of Mental Health Service in England
Figure 7.2 helps show an overview of the different teams present in mental health services.

NHS Mental Health Implementation Plan 2019
NHS England, and the government, have recognised the importance of *parity of esteem* between physical and mental health care. To this end, the Mental Health Implementation Plan set out several goals to be achieved by 2023/24 including:
- 100% coverage of a 24/7 mental health crisis service for children and young people
- 390,000 adults who have SMIs are to receive full physical health checks per year
- 55,000 are to have access to Individual Placement and Support (IPS) plans
- Older adults will have consistent access to mental health support
- Suicide prevention, and bereavement support, programmes to exist in all local areas.

Parity of Esteem
Patients with SMIs die up to 20 years earlier than the general UK population. Parity of esteem states that mental healthcare should be treated as equal to physical healthcare in terms of funding and resources allocation. The 'Five-year Forward View for Mental Health 2016' was part of the way that NHS tried to achieve parity, by embedding it into all systems. The Mental Health Implementation Plan 2019 (above) has further emphasised parity.

Current Barriers
Various areas need to be addressed to achieve parity, these areas include:
- Funding
- Ambition, Access and Targets
- Workforce
- Prevention.

Funding
Over recent years, the healthcare budget has increased, and the percentage spent on mental health services has also increased - but not sufficiently to achieve complete parity of esteem. Without further funding, general practices will not be able to employ mental health professionals, to support the 9 out of 10 people with mental illnesses who are cared for in primary care.

Access, Ambition and Targets
To achieve equal access, targets must be set and there needs to be ambition. For this reason, the NHS set targets for mental health in April 2015 for the first time. This stated that, by April 2016, 75% of people with common mental illnesses were to receive IAPT treatment within 6 weeks of referral, and 95% of people within 18 weeks; and for those having their first episode of psychosis, 50% were to receive NICE-recommended treatments within 2 weeks of referral. These targets have subsequently been tightened.

From August 2015, there has also been a standard for eating disorders. This is that 95% of children and young people (up to the age of 19 years), referred for assessment or treatment for an eating disorder, should receive NICE-approved treatment - within 1 week if the case is urgent, and 4 weeks if the case is non-urgent. Also, by 2020/21, another ambition of the 'Five-year Forward View for Mental Health' was to reduce the suicide rate by 10%.

Workforce
In 2017 Health Education England published 'Stepping Forward to 2020/21, a Mental Health Workforce Plan for England'; whilst the Royal College of Psychiatrists developed a campaign called 'Choose Psychiatry', to address the psychiatry recruitment and retention crisis.

Legal Aspects of Mental Health Care
Mental Health Act (MHA) 1983
The MHA is a legal framework by which patients who show signs of mental illness can be assessed; and if necessary, detained in hospital against their will (for reasons of their health, safety or the safety of others). This is called a 'section' and requires two doctors to carry out.

An application for compulsory 'admission for assessment' (Section 2) can be made on the following grounds:
- The patient is suffering from a mental disorder of degree or nature that warrants admission to a hospital
- It is necessary for the interests of the patient's own health, safety or the safety of others.

An application for compulsory 'admission for treatment' (Section 3) can be made on the following grounds:
- The patient is suffering from a mental disorder of degree or nature that warrants treatment in a hospital
- If it is necessary for the patient's own health and safety, or the safety of others, the patient can receive treatment which otherwise could not be given without detention
- Appropriate treatment is available.

'Admission for assessment' is for up to 28 days for assessment (and treatment). This is normal for those who don't have an established diagnosis. The 'admission for treatment' is for up to 6 months of treatment, for people with an established diagnosis.

Patients have legal rights when they have been detained under the MHA, as does their nearest relative. They can appeal against their section and have the right to legal representation to do so.

An application for detention under the MHA is made by an approved mental health professional (AMHP). An AMHP is someone who has specialist training to carry out duties under the MHA. In most circumstances, this will be a social worker or a mental health nurse. To make an application, the AMHP needs recommendations from two registered medical practitioners, at least one who needs to be approved under Section 12 of the MHA.

However, the AMHP can decide not to make the application, despite the two doctors' recommendations for the patient to be detained. The AMHP is therefore a safeguard that looks for the least restrictive method to treat the patient safely. This may mean the patient is not detained and instead has home treatment from the Mental Health Crisis Team.

Mental Capacity Act (MCA) 2005
This is a legal framework to decide on what care and treatment would be in the best interests of a patient who lacks capacity; the aim being to use the least restrictive method to achieve the result. Family and friends may be consulted to help decide what would be in the person's best interest. However, they would not legally be able to decide for the patient, unless they had been appointed as a 'lasting power of attorney'.

The key principles of the MCA are:
1. Assume a person has capacity unless proven otherwise
2. All practicable measures should be taken to help a person who lacks capacity, to gain capacity to make the decision (an individual has the right to be supported when deciding for themselves)
3. Any decision made should be in the best interest of the patient
4. Use the least restrictive method to carry out the necessary actions.

The Act recognises that a patient who lacks the capacity to decide for themselves is unable to, either:
1. Understand the relevant information to make a decision; or,
2. Retain the information; or,
3. Weigh up in the balance of the information that they are given; or,
4. Communicate their decision (by talking, sign language or any other means of communications).

If an individual is younger than 16, the Children's Act 1989 is the legal framework used.

Holding Powers
There are several holding powers that can be used for people who are inpatients (on mental health or physical health wards). If staff are concerned regarding a patient's mental health (and feel it is not safe for them to leave the ward), the medical doctor in charge of the patient's care can use 'Section 5(2)' to hold the patient for up to 72 hours (to arrange for a mental health act assessment). If the doctor is not immediately available, nursing staff can use 'holding Section 5(4)' for 6 hours, whilst assessment by a doctor is being arranged.

Deprivation of Liberty Safeguard (DoLS)
DoLS are a part of the MCA and can only be used in England and Wales. A DoLS authorisation, from the local authority, is required if a patient lacks capacity and needs to be deprived of their liberty in a care home or a hospital. This is usually to provide necessary treatment or to keep the patient safe.

Lasting Power of Attorney (LPA)
An LPA is when someone appoints one or more people to help make decisions on their behalf, should they later lose the capacity to do so. There are two types:
1. Health and Welfare
2. Property and Financial Affairs.

A person with LPA for health and welfare has the power to make decisions on things such as medical care, decisions regarding care home placement and life-sustaining treatments. An LPA for property and financial affairs has the power to make decisions regarding the person's money and property. This can include functions such as paying bills and selling property.

The Court of Protection
This department makes decisions on financial, and welfare matters in cases where a person lacks capacity and has no LPA.
They have legal powers to:
- Decide whether a person has capacity
- Appoint deputies for those who lack capacity in the long-term
- Grant permission to someone to make a one-off decision on behalf of someone else
- Deal with urgent/emergency applications of decision making on behalf of someone else
- Make decisions on LPAs and consider any outstanding objections regarding their registration
- Consider applications for statutory wills and gifts
- Make decisions on DoLS under the MCA.

Prevention

For mental health, like physical, prevention is better than treatment. For this reason, the NHS Long Term Plan 2019 service goals include preventing or delaying admission, care plan initiation and support provision. It also seeks to implement a revised integrated model of primary and community mental health care.

Perinatal mental health care services will increase their accessibility. And childrens' mental health services will expand their community-based support; such that by 2023/24, an additional 345,000 0–25 year olds will gain access to NHS-funded services.

Prevention of obesity, smoking and alcohol abuse is another focus of the NHS Long Term Plan, as people with mental illnesses are likely to be obese, smoke and drink alcohol. This will be done by increasing the accessibility to weight management services within primary care; particularly for those who have a BMI of 30+, and/or been diagnosed with type 2 diabetes or hypertension. In terms of alcohol abuse, the establishment of Alcohol Care Teams should help reduce attendance to emergency departments.

Further reading

British Medical Association: Beyond parity of esteem – Achieving parity of resource, access and outcome for mental health in England.

https://www.bma.org.uk/media/2099/mental-health-parity-of-esteem-report-jan-2020-2.pdf

Health and Safety Executive: Work-related Stress, Depression or Anxiety Statistics in Great Britain 2019.

https://www.hse.gov.uk/statistics/lfs/index.htm

Mental health and wellbeing in England: Adult Psychiatric Morbidity Survey 2014. https://digital.nhs.uk/data-and-information/publications/statistical/adult-psychiatric-morbidity-survey/adult-psychiatric-morbidity-survey-survey-of-mental-health-and-wellbeing-england-2014

NHS Blog on the achievements and challenges of IAPT.

https://www.england.nhs.uk/blog/iapt-at-10-achievements-and-challenges/

NHS Mental Health Implementation Plan 2019/20 – 2023/24.

https://www.longtermplan.nhs.uk/wp-content/uploads/2019/07/nhs-mental-health-implementation-plan-2019-20-2023-24.pdf

Chapter 8

Public Health

"Healthcare is vital to all of us some of the time, but public health is vital to all of us all of the time." Everett Koop. Former United States Surgeon General.

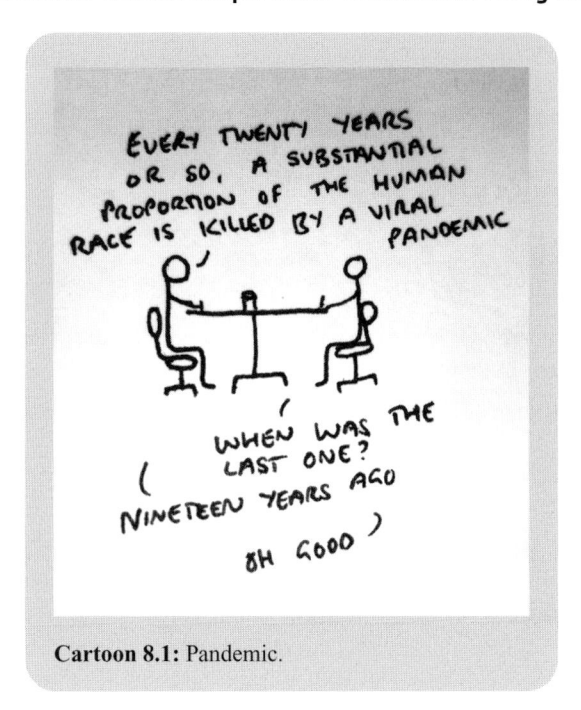

Cartoon 8.1: Pandemic.

Introduction
Most of the major advances in healthcare over the last 200 years have been in public health. Why? (1) It focuses on prevention rather than treatment. And (2), the efficacy of many modern medical treatments is over-stated, e.g. a drug is often said to be effective if it benefits one in 50 users.

Public health (PH) is defined by the World Health Organisation (WHO) as,

"the art and science of preventing disease, prolonging life and promoting health through the organized efforts of society".

PH covers both physical and mental health and wellbeing. There are three key pillars of public health: *health protection, health promotion* and *healthcare public health*.

An organisation called Public Health England (PHE) was responsible for public health in England, but was relaunched in 2021 as the UK Health Security Agency (UKHSA).

Health Protection

Health protection focuses on protecting the public from environmental and biological threats such as radiation, infectious diseases and chemical hazards. It also provides guidance on emergency response procedures and migrant health - and is responsible for immunisation.

It is the duty of medical practitioners and laboratories in the UK to notify the health protection team of suspected cases of 'notifiable diseases', as specified in the Notifications of Infectious Diseases (NOIDS) list. The aim is to rapidly detect and control possible outbreaks of disease, e.g. Swine Flu, Severe Acute Respiratory Syndrome (SARS), C19, Measles and food poisoning.

The occurrence of these diseases and organisms are compiled into weekly reports, to monitor both local and national trends, and track and predict outbreaks. Then appropriate action can be taken to control such outbreaks, as seen with the C19 pandemic.

Pandemics and Epidemics
Influenza A

Influenza A virus subtype H1N1 (or 'Swine Flu') entered the UK from Mexico in April 2009. From two cases in Scotland, 85,000 people were thought to have been affected by mid-July - including 29 confirmed deaths. England's Chief Medical Officer (CMO) at the time, Professor Sir Liam Donaldson, predicted a worst-case scenario of 65,000 deaths, with a minimum death toll of 3,100.

Fortunately, the UK had been preparing for an influenza pandemic since 2005, following the 'Avian Influenza' ('Bird Flu') viral pandemic in 2003; and had 33.5 million units of the antiviral agents Tamiflu® (oseltamivir) and Relenza® (zanamivir) ready. Following the deaths in Mexico from the Swine Flu epidemic, and WHO raising the alert to level 4, this was increased to 50 million units (enough to cover 80% of the population).

With statistics showing Swine Flu predominantly affected 5-14 year olds, government officials were quick to close schools following confirmed cases (the first being in Devon in April). Tamiflu® (oseltamivir) and Relenza® (zanamivir) were given to suspected cases awaiting diagnostic confirmation. Contact tracing was set up and close contacts were given antivirals as a precautionary measure, even if asymptomatic. In addition, schools were closed nationwide.

A vaccine for H1N1, known as 'Pandemrix', was developed by pharmaceutical company GlaxoSmithKline in 2006 but not licenced for use in the UK until 2009. By mid-June there was enough procured to treat the entire UK population, with a large-scale vaccination programme running by October.

A year after the first two cases, the UK was back to normal with the vaccination programme wound up. GPs stopped prescribing antivirals for symptomatic patients, the Swine Flu Information Line was closed, and flu treatment went back to 'business as usual'. In total, the UK saw 27,464 confirmed cases with 457 deaths. Worldwide estimates were that 700 million to 1.4 billion were infected, and 284,000 people died.

Severe Acute Respiratory Syndrome (SARS)
SARS originated in China in 2002 and came to the UK in 2003. Caused by the coronavirus SARS-CoV-1 virus, over 8,000 were infected worldwide, and at least 774 died. By March 2003, there were 761 cases of SARS in 15 countries and Britain saw its four confirmed cases. The UK SARS taskforce was formed. Travellers coming into the UK were assessed as to whether they had travelled from 'high-risk' areas, and followed up with samples collected for SARS-CoV antibodies. Early detection was vital in minimising SARS cases in the UK.

COVID-19
SARS-CoV-2, more commonly known as COVID-19 (C19), swept the UK from January 2020 as part of a worldwide pandemic. Cases increased rapidly during March and the government established a 'COVID action plan' with anyone showing symptoms being asked to self-isolate for seven days; which was quickly followed with advice against foreign travel, and meeting in public places. The government also insisted people worked from home if possible, and introduced 'social distancing' (keeping at least two metres away from other people).

Surgical operations were cancelled, and schools, pubs, restaurants and gyms were closed. On 23 March, the UK initiated a nationwide 'lockdown' following total deaths rising to 1,019 with a daily death toll of 100 people. During lockdown the public had to stay at home, only leaving to collect essentials such as food and medicines. Initially only supposed to last for three weeks, the lockdown lasted three months, as new cases and deaths continued to rise. Lockdown was officially lifted on 4 July, but strict C19 guidelines were put in place. Wearing face coverings became a legal requirement in public places in late July - as rules adapted in response to infection rates.

After a second wave of the virus, a second national lockdown for four weeks (this time with schools open) ran from 5 November to 2 December. The second wave merged with a third wave, fuelled by a more infectious variant. The country went back into national lockdown (with schools closed) on 5 January 2021. A slow relaxation of the third lockdown started on 8 March when schools returned, and people were allowed to meet one other person outside. The process ended on the 19 of July 2021, which was declared 'Freedom Day', when most C19 restrictions were lifted. By then, a significant proportion of the adult population had been vaccinated.[18]

Immunisation
The UK has a routine immunisation programme offered to all babies, operated by the NHS. This means by the time any infant is 1-year old, they will have been immunised against: diphtheria, tetanus, pertussis (whooping cough), polio, haemophilus influenzae type b (Hib), hepatitis B, meningococcal group B (MenB) and C (MenC) bacteria, rotavirus gastroenteritis, pneumococcal bacteria (13 serotypes), measles, mumps and rubella (German measles). It is estimated vaccines prevent 3 million deaths worldwide annually.

---

18. 43.5 million people (80.1% of the adult population) had received both vaccines by the 8 September 2021 'https://coronavirus.data.gov.uk/details/vaccinations'

And in the UK, many of these previously common diseases have either disappeared or are now rare (or very rare).

Measles was considered eradicated in the UK by the World Health Organisation in 2017; and although this is no longer the case, there has been a 99.9% reduction in measles cases since the vaccines were introduced. Similarly, diphtheria cases saw a 99.9% reduction in cases with only four deaths attributed to diphtheria in the last 20 years. In 2019, there were only four cases of tetanus. The vaccination programme has also resulted in the extinction of some diseases such as Smallpox (which the WHO considers eradicated worldwide) and polio (which has not been seen in the UK since the 80s).

The human papillomavirus (HPV) vaccination programme was introduced for 12-13 year old girls in 2008 before being extended to males in 2019. HPV is a sexually transmitted virus that comes in over 100 forms. Importantly HPV16 and 18 cause up to 80% of cervical cancers, whereas HPV 6 and 11 cause 90% of genital warts. Since the introduction of routine vaccination, HPV cases had dropped by 86% in 2018, reducing pre-cancerous cervical disease by up to 71%. Diagnoses of genital warts have declined by 90% in 15-17 year old girls, and by 70% in 15-17 year old boys.

Cervical cancer is currently the most common cancer for women under 35 years in the UK, killing 850 a year. With vaccination, the numbers are expected to fall by a further 36% in women aged 25-29 years, and 28% in those aged 30-34 years, by 2036-40.

Air, Water and the Environment

Due to Britain's industrial history, many areas of land were previously factories, mills and mines. In those places, industry created a lot of waste products; amongst them heavy metals (such as arsenic, cadmium and lead), oils and tars, chemical substances and preparations (like solvents), gases, asbestos and radioactive substances.

Local councils will classify land based on the risk of being contaminated, with 'Category 1' being a significant risk to health, and 'Category 4' being an acceptable low risk. They will then take soil samples, test for relevant chemicals and toxicity of the samples. Once this testing has been completed, a risk assessment is completed to guide appropriate action.

For water, there are only legal requirements related to the quality of *drinking* water, with guidance documents only pertaining to water maintenance systems (such as pools, heaters, dialysis, etc.). Water samples are examined for Coliform bacteria, Escherichia coli, Pseudomonas aeruginosa, Aerobic Colony Counts, environmental Mycobacteria, Legionella, Endotoxin and various chemical contaminants. Water temperature control must also be assessed to help explain any microbiological issues.

Air pollutants can affect different organs and systems such as the heart and lungs. Air pollutants have been linked to low birth weight, and delayed lung development in children. In middle and later life, air pollutants can lead to lung problems (e.g. cancers and chronic obstructive pulmonary disease), strokes, heart attacks, and even diabetes. In addition, long-term air pollutant exposure can result in asthma, regardless of age; and has also been linked to dementia.

In 2010, the Environment Audit Committee stated the health cost of air pollution was likely to be £8-20 billion per year. It has been estimated that long term exposure to air pollutants causes 28,000 to 36,000 deaths a year; and lowering fine air particulate by 1ug/m^3 could prevent around 50,900 cases of coronary heart disease, 16,500 strokes, 9,300 cases of asthma and 4,200 lung cancers over an 18-year period.

There are many air pollutants linked to health, including: particulate matter (PM), nitrogen dioxide (NO_2), sulphur dioxide (SO_2), ammonia (NH_3), ozone (O_3), carbon monoxide (CO), and Non-Methane Volatile Organic Compounds (NMVOCs). PM is the general term given to a complex mixture of solid and liquid particles of varying sizes, shapes, and composition. The different sizes of PM affect the body in different ways; with larger PM being linked to problems in the nose and throat, and smaller PM linked to problems deeper in the lung.

NO_2 is a gas produced by combustion processes, such as in car engines, energy production and industrial processes. In the short-term, it causes inflammation and irritation of the airways, leading to cough and shortness of breath. Exposure in children affects lung development.

NMVOCs come from a wide variety of products and processes and is a significant component of indoor air pollution from household products. NMVOCs react with NO_2 to form O_3 (ozone), the gas usually found natural in the Earth's upper atmosphere. When produced at ground level, O_3 has an impact on respiratory and cardiovascular health. SO_2 and NH_3 are gases that can react with other chemicals to form acids and cause environmental damage. Additionally, NH_3 can react with acid gases, such as sulphuric and nitric acid, to form secondary PM.

Health Promotion

Health promotion is concerned with helping people to make better health related choices. It aims to improve health by addressing both individual, and collective,

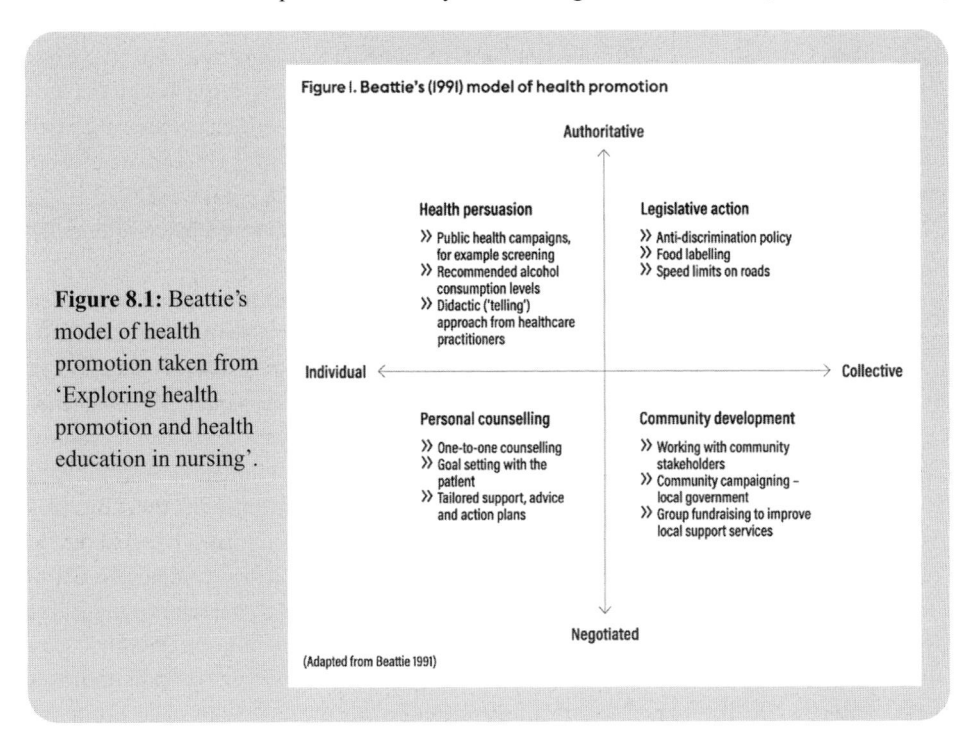

Figure 8.1: Beattie's model of health promotion taken from 'Exploring health promotion and health education in nursing'.

Figure I. Beattie's (1991) model of health promotion

Authoritative

Health persuasion
>> Public health campaigns, for example screening
>> Recommended alcohol consumption levels
>> Didactic ('telling') approach from healthcare practitioners

Legislative action
>> Anti-discrimination policy
>> Food labelling
>> Speed limits on roads

Individual ←→ Collective

Personal counselling
>> One-to-one counselling
>> Goal setting with the patient
>> Tailored support, advice and action plans

Community development
>> Working with community stakeholders
>> Community campaigning – local government
>> Group fundraising to improve local support services

Negotiated

(Adapted from Beattie 1991)

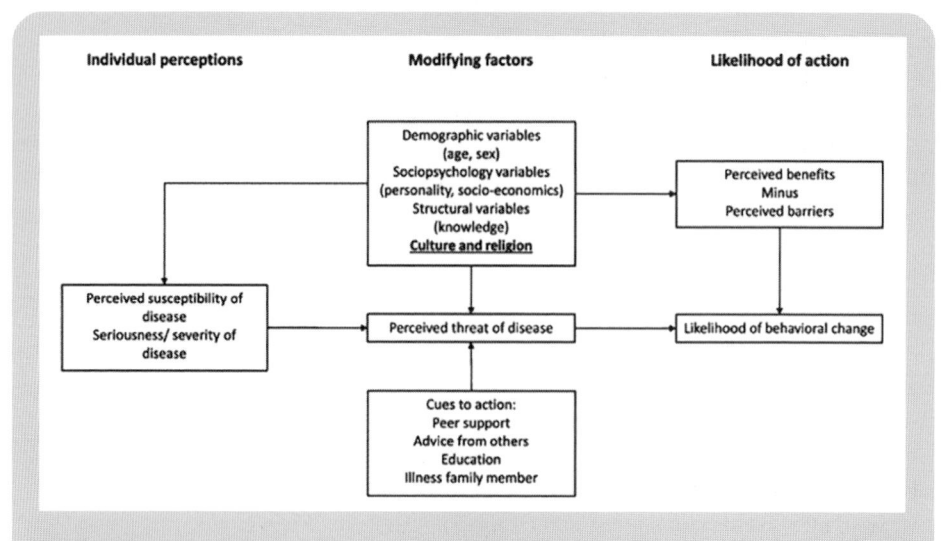

Figure 8.2: Hochbaum, Rosenstock and Kegels' health belief model taken from 'The Health Belief model'.

responsibility. These strategies are based on one of two health models: Beattie's model of health promotion (Figure 8.1) and Hochbaum, Rosenstock and Kegels' health belief model (Figure 8.2).

Individual Basis

Focusing on an individual aspect of health, guides people to make better health choices. We see this regularly on TV, in the news or in our GP surgery - often in the form of a campaign. Think of the 'Change4life' campaign (to tackle obesity), 'Smokefree NHS', and the 'F.A.S.T.' campaign (to recognise strokes early).

Change4life was introduced in 2009 focusing on preventing weight *gain,* rather than targeting weight loss, via a large-scale social media campaign. Its primary focus was families, especially those with children under 11 years. Its conception came after it was recorded in 2007 that a quarter of adults were obese, and 65% of men and 56% of women were overweight. The campaign focused on the risks of obesity and its health consequences; and then promoted the benefits of exercise and a healthier diet. Research done prior to the campaign revealed families, whilst knowing childhood obesity was a problem, did not consider obesity to be their major issue. They would under-estimate food consumption and over-estimate the amount of exercise they performed.

The campaign unfolded in five phases, the first began by linking weight gain with illness and reduced life expectancy, followed by phase two which involved making the issues personal. It shifted the focus to the individual's own family by posing the question: 'how are the kids?'. Phase three defined the behaviours that needed changing and condensed them into eight behaviours to change:

1. Reducing sugar intake ('Sugar Swaps')
2. Increasing consumption of fruit and vegetables ('5 A Day')
3. Having structured meals, especially breakfast ('Meal Time')
4. Reducing unhealthy snacking ('Snack Check')
5. Reducing portion size ('Me Size Meals')
6. Reducing fat consumption ('Cut Back Fat')
7. 60 minutes of moderate intensity activity ('60 Active Minutes')
8. Reducing sedentary behaviour ('Up & About').

Phase four focused on showing that change was achievable using personal stories of change in addition to local events to inspire change. The final phase was to support those committed to changing. Campaign materials were readily available, delivered out to families and accessible online. The campaign was successful, with 413,466 families signing up and 44,833 families continuing their involvement six months on.

'Smokefree NHS' was started by PHE in 2016, and had 3 aims:
- All frontline medical staff should discuss smoking with patients
- Every smoker using NHS services is offered stop smoking support on site or referred to a local service
- Everyone understands there is 'no smoking' on NHS premises.

The NHS free smoking cessation service utilises one-to-one, and group stop smoking sessions run at local GP surgeries, pharmacies, high-street shops and even a mobile bus clinic. In addition, the NHS promotes several 'stop smoking aids' such as nicotine replacement products (including patches, gum, lozenges, inhalators and mouth and nasal sprays), and

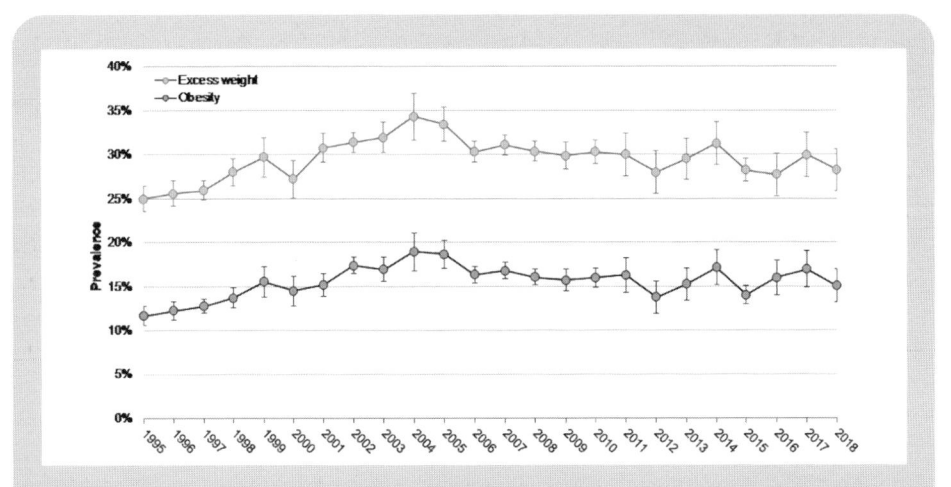

Figure 8.3: Since 2009, when Change4life was introduced, rates of excess weight and obesity and children has been variable. Graph taken from 'Patterns and trends in child obesity by Public Health England'.

stop smoking tablets. Following the sessions, the NHS aims to prevent relapse with regular contact for the first four weeks, replace stop smoking aids and monitor carbon monoxide.

The campaign has been shown to be effective, with those who participate being four times more likely to quit. The adult smoking rate in England continues to decline annually, and in 2017, 6.1 million (14.9%) adults in England smoked. Current predictions forecast a reduction to between 8.5% and 11.7% by 2023, and a smoke free society by 2030.

Collective Basis

Health can be improved with legislation to impose large scale changes, e.g. the 'sugar tax', drink driving legislation and fluoridisation of drinking water.

The 'sugar tax', also known as the soft drinks industry levy (SDIL), was brought into effect in 2018 to reduce childhood obesity. The SDIL means soft drink manufacturers pay a surcharge on any beverage containing more than 8g of sugar. The benefits of these extra charges are two-fold: first soft drinks are altered to contain less sugar; and, second, the companies refusing to change, will pay additional tax. In the two years leading up to the introduction of the SDIL, 50% of soft drink manufacturers reduced the sugar content in their drinks - equivalent to 45 million kilograms of sugar annually.

In addition to lifestyle change, the aim of health promotion is to reduce social and economic inequalities as outlined by Dahlgren and Whitehead in 1991 (Figure 4). This includes issues such as school meals, employment and living standards. The importance of addressing social inequality was explicitly highlighted in the Black Report in 1980, which confirmed social class health inequalities in overall mortality (and for most causes

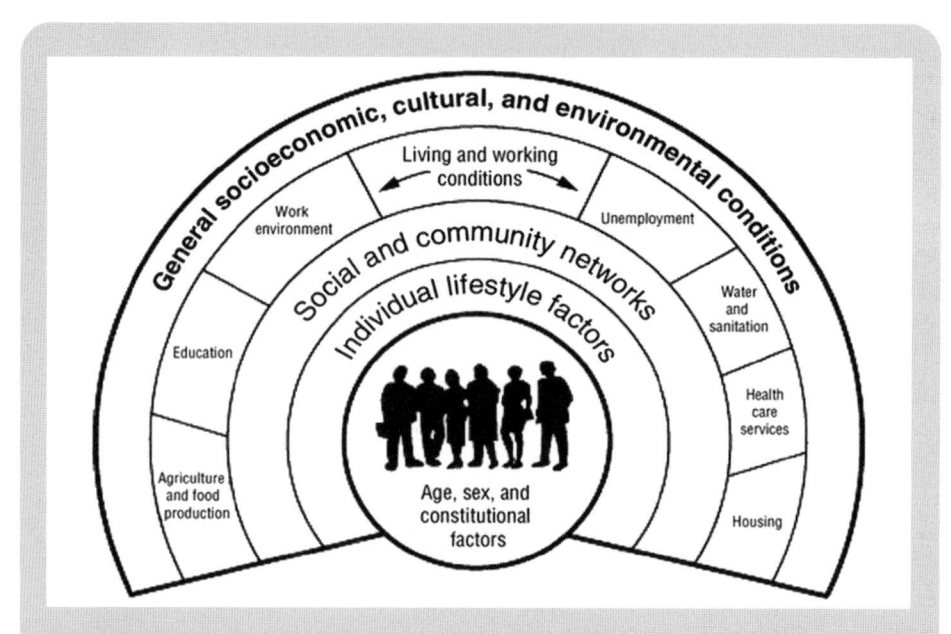

Figure 8.4: Dahlgren and Whitehead's health rainbow outlining the different components that contribute to an individual's health.

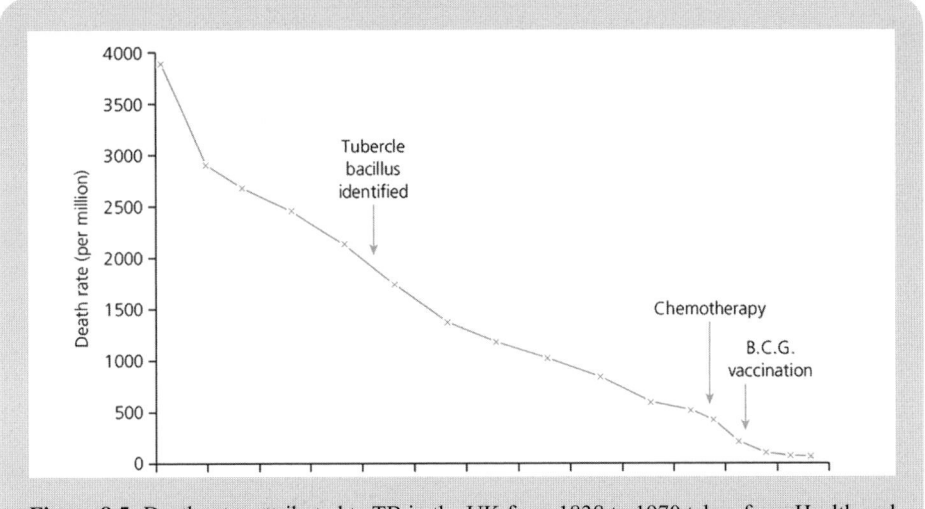

Figure 8.5: Death rates attributed to TB in the UK from 1838 to 1970 taken from Health and Health Policy (2012).

of death) - and showed health inequalities were widening. Health promotion in this regard, focuses on how our environment, employment and income have an effect on health; for example, how living conditions can impact the spread of disease (e.g. tuberculosis), and how unemployment leads to an inability to afford a healthier diet.

Tuberculosis
Tuberculosis (TB) is a good example of a 'social disease'. It is a chronic bacterial infection spread through inhaling tiny droplets from the coughs or sneezes of an infected person. Its risk of spread increases with close contact especially in dark, poorly ventilated and overcrowded spaces. Due to its increased ability to spread in overcrowded spaces, TB is more common in deprived areas where housing conditions are poorer. In 2015, the rate of TB was 20.5 per 100,000 in the 10% of the population living in the most deprived areas; compared with only 3.6 per 100,000 in the 10% of the population living in the least deprived areas. C19 has behaved in similar ways.

TB is therefore a disease of inequality affecting disproportionate numbers of ethnic minorities, migrants, prisoners, and people who are homeless or use recreational drugs. To tackle this inequality, steps are being taken, including tackling the stigma around TB and raising awareness; especially among healthcare professionals working in high prevalence areas.

There is also an emphasis on early diagnosis which is associated with better outcomes at less cost. The work to reduce TB rates is co-ordinated by a collaboration of local authorities, Clinical Commissioning Groups (CCGs), TB Control Boards and TB Clinical Teams.

Healthcare Public Health
Healthcare public health is about ensuring health services are as effective, efficient and equally accessible, as possible. It covers more than just funding hospital care or general practice.

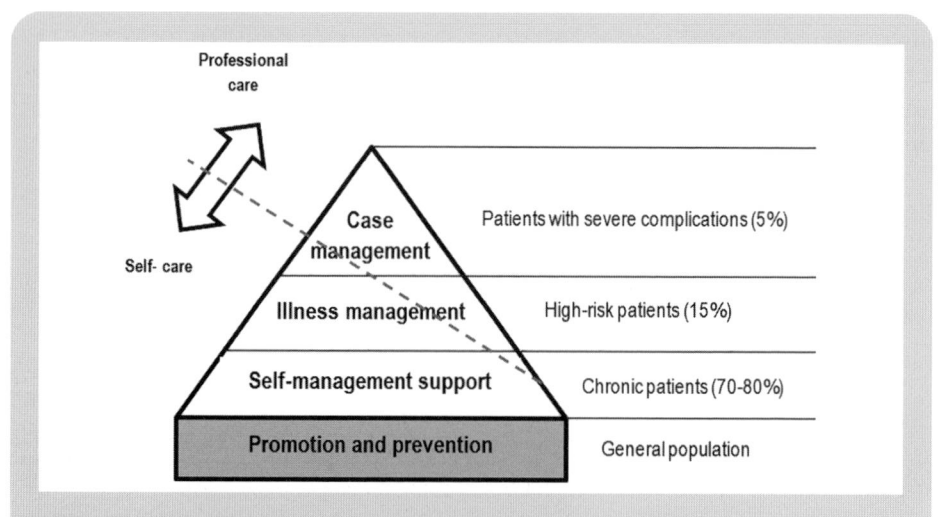

Figure 8.6: The 'Kaiser Pyramid Care Model' taken from 'Integrated care models: an overview'. People require more care and better access to resources as you move up the pyramid.

Need and Supply

It is important to balance the health needs of society and patient groups with the availability of NHS care. The small percentage of the population with more severe and complex conditions, however, require more resources than those who are generally well (Figure 8.6).

Need, in this case, does not necessarily mean 'need for healthcare'. A person may need healthcare but not be ill (as with preventative medicine) or may be ill but require no medical care (such as when medicine may be ineffective). Instead, need is better defined as the 'capacity to benefit from services', which relies on access, equity and equality.'

Access to Healthcare

Access to healthcare is the ability for an individual to get the treatment they need. It is comprised of 3 parts: physical access, timely access and choice.

Physical Access

This can be limited by several factors such as availability of services, geographical location, disability, age, gender, language, culture, knowledge of services, and fear. Areas of higher deprivation may not have the resources to provide services. Similarly, if a patient is too far away (geographically) from the services they need, and cannot travel or afford to travel, their physical access is limited.

People living with disabilities need to be accommodated in service design and provision, otherwise they potentially lose access to services, e.g. the need for ramps, or special equipment and specialised staff.

Language and cultural differences are a problem facing immigrants, who may struggle to obtain the care they need; perhaps through fear relating to their uncertain migration status and concerns regarding deportation. Fear of being judged can also prevent people who use drugs and alcohol, the homeless, sex workers and the LGBTQ+ community from seeking care. It is our duty, as a health professional, not to be concerned with the origins, gender or behaviours of a person that needs our help.

Timely Access
This refers to whether patients can be seen when needed and concerns appointment availability, waiting times and out-of-hours services.

Choice
The idea of 'choice' began in the early 2000s in the Blair/Brown era. It is controversial as many argue it was (and is) a vote winner but not actually a real choice, e.g. in 2000 'walk-in centres' started as an alternative to general practice with no appointment or registration needed. It was a real choice. But in 2006 it became mandatory for a patient to be given a choice of three 'providers' (hospitals) if they needed to see a specialist. However often one was local, one 50 miles away and one 200 miles away!

Also patients may simply lack the information regarding services they are entitled to, e.g. there are many names for what we think of as a 'walk-in centre', such as Urgent Care Centre (UCC), and Minor Injury Unit (MIU). Such acronyms confuse people who are not sure where to go and so default to the emergency department (ED).

Finally, it is important to note, despite advances in the education of society, the average reading ability of an adult in the UK population is that of a 9-year old. Furthermore, according to the National Literacy Trust, 16% of adults in the UK are considered 'functionally illiterate'. Thus public health information must always be kept simple (the 'KISS' principle = 'keep it simple, stupid').

Equity and Equality in Healthcare
Equity involves addressing differences between groups within a population, so all groups have the same level of access to a service. This is achieved by unevenly distributing resources to those with more need - so different groups get more or less of something, depending on their needs, and a universal standard is met.

In contrast, *equality* is when people are treated the same, meaning everyone has the same access to resources. Equality is important within a group. So every member of that group has the exact same resources. If this were applied between groups, social inequalities based on wealth, power, or prestige would persist - hence the need for equity.

Distributive Justice
Distributive justice relates to equality and is centred on distributing resources fairly by making them equal regardless of age, sex, quality of life, socioeconomic status and race. It is built on two concepts: 'utilitarianism' and the 'veil of ignorance'. Utilitarianism, founded in the 18th Century by Jeremy Bentham, is described as,

"the greatest good for the greatest number";

and is about maximising the amount of good done for the greatest number of people. Utilitarianism is commonly illustrated using the 'trolley thought experiment': would you redirect a trolley car (a tram) to hit one person to prevent it hitting five people? In the eyes of a utilitarian, five people benefit from your decision to redirect the trolley; and it is therefore the correct and most ethical option (despite you being directly responsible for the death of one person).

The 'veil of ignorance' was popularised by John Rawls in 1971. The 'veil' questions how decision-makers make decisions; i.e. (1) do they first have the information to know the consequence of their choice; and (2) know if the choice will leave them in the group that will benefit most from their decision? Neither may be true. Therefore, the decision-maker should choose an option that benefits all groups. For example, if there is a vaccine for a disease only 50% of a group will die of, and the decision-maker does not know which group they are in, they will vaccinate everyone.

When the two concepts of utilitarianism and the veil of ignorance are combined, it is logical that resources should be allocated in a way that benefits the greatest number of people, regardless which groups they are a part of.

Procedural Justice

Procedural justice, in contrast, concerns itself with whether decisions are considered in a just and fair way. It is built on six characteristics: accuracy, consistency, impartiality, reversibility, transparency and voice. It involves listening to the opinions of the public before making decisions; and those decisions are then made openly and honestly (whilst addressing the concerns raised). The decision then needs to be applied consistently across similar problems, and should be made without being affected by the decision-maker's own thoughts and feelings. This concept leads to resources being distributed based on equity, and by making decisions based on the concerns of individual groups - as opposed to blanket decisions to benefit the most people.

Use of Resources

Decisions are not only made based on equality or equity. As resources are limited, the most efficient use of resources must be considered to maximise efficacy whilst limiting expenditure. Resources are limited because the *need for healthcare is unlimited*. So societies must ration healthcare investment; to make sure other aspects of society (defence, law and order, transport, education, etc.) have their share of taxation.

Thus someone must make the decision based on either the greatest benefit from a set amount of resource, or the lowest resource requirement for set level of benefit. An inefficient healthcare service would lead to the public not having access to the resources they need, receiving below par care, not trusting the system, or becoming unwilling to use the health service (especially if it appeared to be wasteful).

Health systems therefore need to ensure they are accessible, efficient and effective. This is achieved through regular monitoring, evaluation, auditing and investigating *outliers*. Audits allow a service to see what it does well, what it does less well, and what changes can be made to improve. By investigating outliers, i.e. those that stray from the norm, it can be determined why this is happening. For example, if a particular hospital was getting more cases of a certain illness than the surrounding hospitals, there could be a range of causes: a unique health issue may exist; an unnecessary initiative to look for work may be taking place; or the disease is not being managed properly and patients are returning.

Data is very important in helping to use resources efficiently and is used at a local level by Clinical Commissioning Groups (CCGs). But they will only make good decisions if they have good data to base these on.

Examples of Major Public Health Initiatives

There have been many successful public health initiatives in the UK, notable among these, have been the campaign to reduce smoking, and introduce a seatbelt law.

Smoking

The link between smoking and cancer was first established in a 1950 UK study by Richard Doll and Tony Bradford Hill. In 1954, they also demonstrated smokers had higher mortality rates than non-smokers. But it was not until 1962, however, that the dangers of smoking entered the mind of the British public with the publication of the Royal College of Physicians' 'Smoking and Health' report; following which doctors were told to warn patients of the risks of smoking. Before this, 70% of men and 40% of women were smokers, with 33% of 'heavy smokers' dying before the age of 65.

Following the publication and government action, tobacco sales dropped. In 1962, 120,840 tonnes of tobacco products were sold. This dropped to 112,990 tonnes by 1972 and continues to fall today. 51% of men were smoking in 1974 when national records on smoking began. In 2011, 19.8% of adults in England were smoking but as of 2019, this number has dropped to 13.9%.

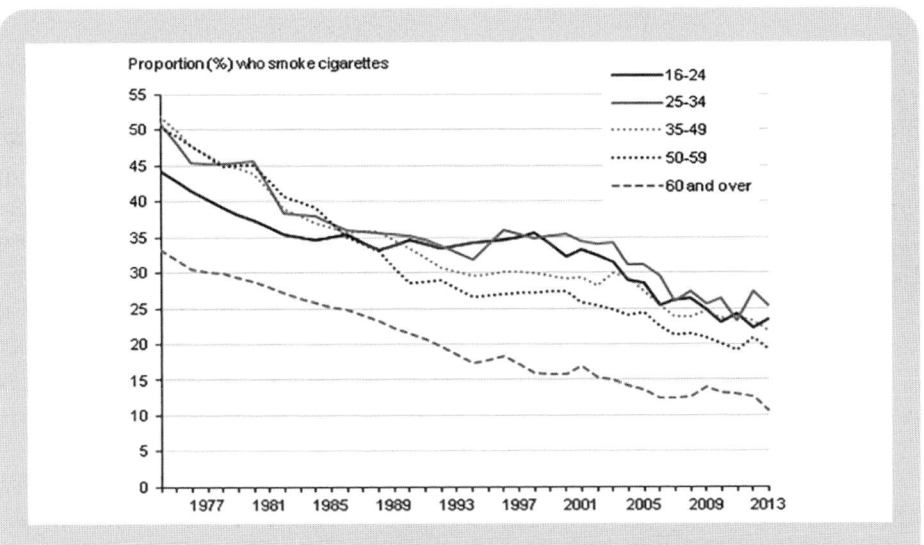

Figure 8.7: The percentage of the English population who smoked between the years of 1974 and 2013, taken from 'publichealthmatters.gov.uk'.

Following the 1962 report, the British government banned TV advertising of cigarettes. Since 1971, it has been a legal requirement to put health warnings on tobacco packaging. The danger of passive smoking was reported for the first time in 1983; and following this, smoking bans began appearing. They first appeared on London Underground trains (1984) before spreading to the entire underground network (1987). A ban in all public places was not proposed until 2002; but it was not until July 2007 that England's smoking ban came into force. The effects were clear, with a 6.3% drop in cigarette sales in England, and air pollution in bars dropping by 93%.

Just one year after the smoking ban in pubs, 1,200 fewer heart attack patients were seen in hospitals. After three years, there was an 18% decrease in children being admitted to hospital with asthma. In addition, the smoking bans have been linked to a lower incidence of stroke and cardiovascular-related hospital admissions and reductions in COPD. With fewer pregnant women smoking, fewer babies were born prematurely or had a low birth weight. Finally, and perhaps most important, the number of deaths related to all smoking-related diseases has also fallen. No medical intervention – whether a medication, operation or new technology - has achieved anything like this improvement in health.

Seatbelts

The law requiring cars to have seat belts put in was passed in 1965. However, having a seat belt and wearing it are very different stories. The push to create a seat belt law was led by *Which?* (a non-profit, goods testing organisation) but it only became a legal requirement to wear a seat belt in the front seat in 1983 (wearing rear seat belts would become compulsory in 1991). The effect was immediate with seat belt wearing rising from 40% to 90%; and the percentage of people dying following motor vehicle accidents dropped by 29%, with a 30% reduction in serious injuries. To put this into perspective, 2,443 people were killed on British roads in 1982. But, following the law change, this number was 1,734; and by 2016, just 816.

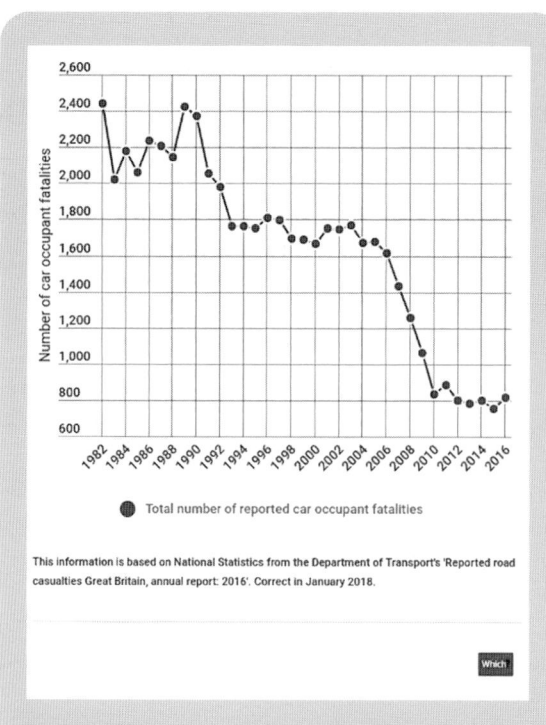

Figure 8.8: The total number of reported car occupant fatalities between 1982 and 2016 taken from 'Which?'.

Public Health Organisation in the UK

Public Health England (PHE) was established in 2013 to provide evidence-based advice and scientific expertise to government, local government, the NHS, industry and the public. The formation of PHE pulled together functions which had previously been the responsibility of many local and national agencies.

PHE was responsible in England for maintaining the health of the nation, reducing health inequality, responding to public health emergencies, protection from environmental hazards, planning for future public health challenges and researching ways to improve public health. It is comprised of four regions and eight local centres. The four regions are North of England, South of England, Midlands and East of England, and London. These were originally meant to work with the four NHS England regions of the same names. In 2019, NHS England's four regions broke up into seven regions, and the public health regions did not, which may be a factor in the UK's poor performance against C19.

Each region has a number of local centres which supervise local public health systems (based at the local council), which provide health protection services, expertise and advice to the local NHS. In addition, the local centres contribute to emergency planning, support local Health and Wellbeing teams, and can provide specialist services such as microbiology laboratory facilities and field epidemiology teams. Each nation of the UK has its own public health organisations. Scotland, Wales and Northern Ireland have Public Health Scotland (PHS), Public Health Wales (PHW) and the Public Health Agency (PHA) respectively.

Partly due to poor performance regarding C19, PHE has been closed down, and a new organisation formed. Performance was little better in the other 3 nations. Hence, on 18 August 2020, the National Institute for Health Protection (NIHP) was established combining PHE with NHS Test and Trace, and the analytical capability of the Joint Biosecurity Centre (JBC) - to cover all four UK nations. This was relaunched as the UK Health Security Agency (UKHSA) in April 2021. It is responsible for:

1. Local health protection teams, to deal with infections and other threats
2. Support and resources for local authorities to manage local outbreaks
3. C19 testing programme and contact tracing
4. The Joint Biosecurity Centre
5. Emergency response and preparedness to deal with the most severe incidents at national and local level
6. The National Infections Services; for example, field services and scientific campuses at Colindale and Porton Down
7. The regional and specialist public health microbiology laboratory network
8. The Centre for Radiation, Chemical and Environmental Hazards
9. Global health security capability
10. The UK public health Rapid Support Team (joint with the London School of Hygiene and Tropical Medicine)
11. Research and knowledge management; working with academic partners through Health Protection Research Units
12. Providing specialist scientific advice on immunisation and countermeasures.

The C19 pandemic has made the UK think about better ways of tackling pandemics, by strengthening health protection systems. For example, in the future, the UKHSA will focus on:
1. Providing evidence and support for national and local government on policy decisions for health improvement
2. Providing expert advice to the NHS and local government, including screening and immunisation programmes
3. Delivering health interventions in the form of social marketing campaigns, to support individuals to take control of their health
4. Undertaking cross-system activity including maintaining the national cancer registry.

There will also be a focus on prevention and improved integration of care.

History of Public Health

The origins of public health in England go back to 1854. During an outbreak of cholera in London's Soho area, John Snow (considered the father of public health medicine and epidemiology) hypothesised that the disease came from a water source contaminated by sewage. The cases of the disease were plotted on a map of the area, which led to one suspected source, a water-pump in Broad Street (Figure 8.9). His claim that cholera was a water-borne disease was correct and, following the removal of the pump handle, cases began to fall.

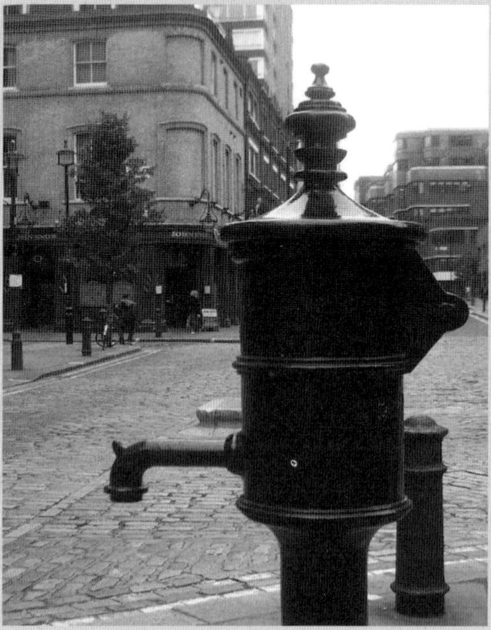

From these humble beginnings, public health and epidemiology were born - leading to the Public Health Acts of 1872 and 1875. It was now compulsory to provide clean water, dispose of sewage and to clean the streets - improving the health of the population. This can be considered the first form of health prevention.

Figure 8.9: The Broad Street Pump in Soho, London.[19]

---

19. Students of public health may want to touch the pump (still in Soho), whilst celebrating public health initiatives in a bar or two.

Early 20th Century

The early 20th Century focused on preventing and treating disease with newly discovered antibiotics and vaccines. Furthermore (often Liberal Party-led) social reforms occurred during this time; with the intention of reducing poverty and improving health for the old, the young, the sick and the unemployed. Between 1906-1914, these reforms saw the introduction of free school meals and medical treatment for children; as well as old age pensions, compulsory health insurance for low-paid workers, and unemployment insurance. Following Lloyd George's National Insurance Act 1911, GPs became responsible for the provision of primary healthcare within a national system funded by the state for the first time (albeit for working males). This system was a key building block of the NHS, and its importance should not be underestimated.

1940s and 50s

Following the Second World War and the formation of the NHS in 1948, the 1950s saw the next major public health initiatives. Smoking was linked to cancer for the first time. The Clean Air Act 1956 was established in response to high mortality rates following the 'Great Smog' of 1952 (which may have killed 12,000 people). 1958 brought in the first vaccination programme. The first Mental Health Act was passed in 1959 (building on previous legislation) and ensured equivalence between mental and physical health.

1960s and 1970s

The 1960s saw a shift from the diseases of poverty to the diseases of affluence. Following further links between smoking and lung health, and cholesterol and heart disease, the emphasis was now on looking after yourself. The public were advised to eat better, stop smoking and exercise more. The 60s also saw the first substantive water fluoridation scheme to improve dental health (Birmingham, 1964); the NHS Family Planning Act 1967 and the Abortion Act 1967. Contraception and family planning advice now had much wider usage, and women were free to decide when they wanted to have a family. This not only changed societal norms but also lowered the risk of financial difficulties in low-income groups.

The Local Authority Social Services Act was put into action in 1970 following the recommendations of the Seebohm Report in 1968. The Act created a framework for local authorities to establish their own social service department. It required every local authority to establish a social services committee, in addition to appointing directors of social services to deliver these functions. The Act also established the Health Secretary of State's authority to provide directions to local authorities on how to use these services. This move highlighted the need for a co-ordinated and comprehensive approach to social care. It allowed local authorities to get better at supporting families, detecting needs within their community and encouraging people to seek help.

The Faculty of Public Health was established in 1972 - the first ever public health professional body in the UK.

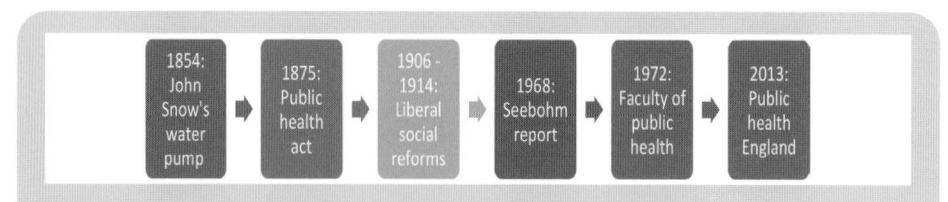

Fig 8.9: A timeline highlighting the major public health events that have occurred since 1854.

Timeline: 1854: John Snow's water pump → 1875: Public health act → 1906-1914: Liberal social reforms → 1968: Seebohm report → 1972: Faculty of public health → 2013: Public health England

1980s and 1990s
Public health in the 80s and 90s focused on health promotion. AIDS campaigns were established, as were breast and cervical screening programmes - and the public were warned about Mad Cow Disease.

2000s and 2010s
The early 2000s saw our focus change to food: with the creation of the Food Standards Agency (FSA) in 2001; the introduction of the '5-a-day' advice regarding fruit and vegetables; and the launch of the 'Change4life campaign' to tackle obesity. The late 2000s also saw the smoking ban (in public places) rolled out nationwide, as well as HPV vaccines for girls aged 12-13 years. The 2010s saw a continued emphasis on health promotion and prevention, with legislation to reduce alcohol and sugar consumption, and the rates of smoking.

2020s
The 2020s have, so far, been dominated by C19, with public health services as important as ever.

Further reading

The British Heart Foundation on the impact of the smoking ban.
https://www.bhf.org.uk/informationsupport/heart-matters-magazine/news/smoking-ban

The Change4Life campaign pages.
https://www.thensmc.com/resources/showcase/change4life

The NHS about why vaccinations are so important.
https://www.nhs.uk/conditions/vaccinations/why-vaccination-is-safe-and-important/

The UK Government pages on the impact of air pollution.
https://www.gov.uk/government/publications/health-matters-air-pollution/health-matters-air-pollution

The UK Health Security Agency page about the impact of the HPV vaccination programme on cervical cancers.
https://ukhsa.blog.gov.uk/2018/06/18/ten-years-on-since-the-start-of-the-hpv-vaccine-programme-what-impact-is-it-having/

World Health Organisation on SARS.
https://www.who.int/ith/diseases/sars/en/

Chapter 9

Research

"Scientific thought is the common heritage of mankind".
Abdus Salam, Pakistani theoretical physicist and Nobel prize winner.

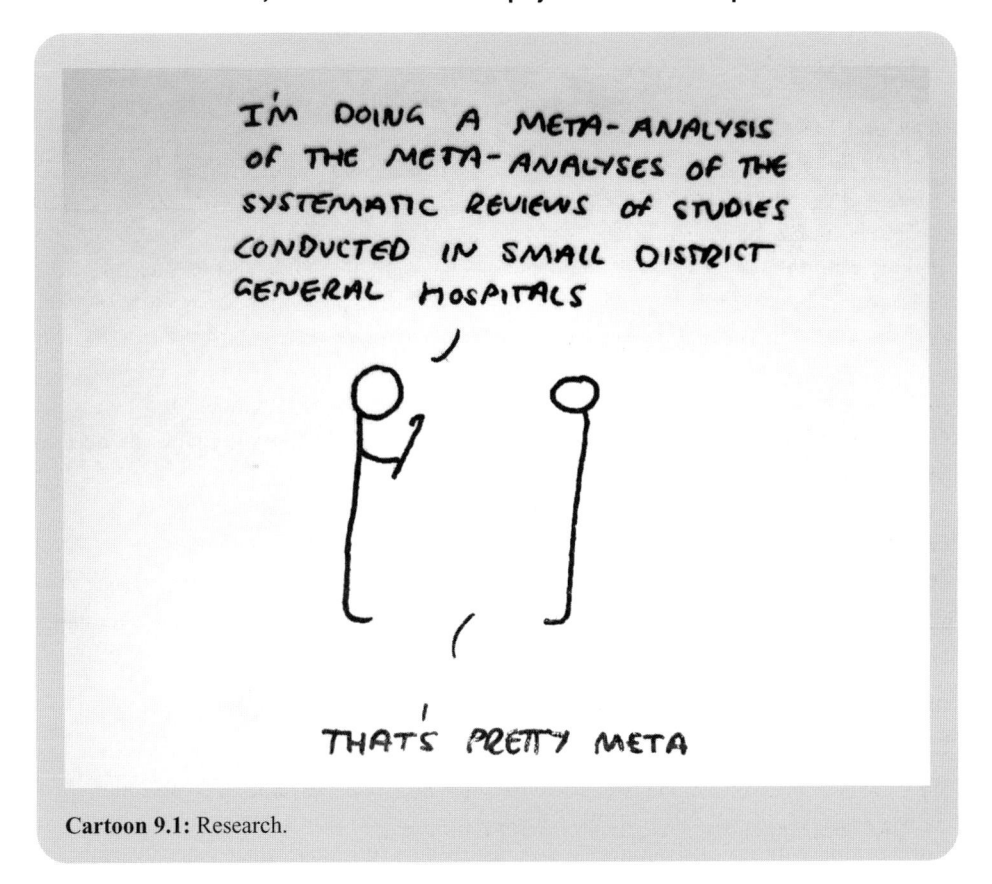

> I'M DOING A META-ANALYSIS OF THE META-ANALYSES OF THE SYSTEMATIC REVIEWS OF STUDIES CONDUCTED IN SMALL DISTRICT GENERAL HOSPITALS
>
> THAT'S PRETTY META

Cartoon 9.1: Research.

Introduction

Research is one of the core values of the NHS. It is also a core need.

The NHS, Health Research Authority (HRA) and National Institute of Health Research (NIHR) collaboratively support research in the UK. The HRA examines ethics, NIHR funds research with the NHS providing the infrastructure.

Dedicated Research and Development (R&D) departments have been established in larger NHS trusts providing support to researchers concerning all aspects of the research

Figure 9.1: NIHR Research Cycle.

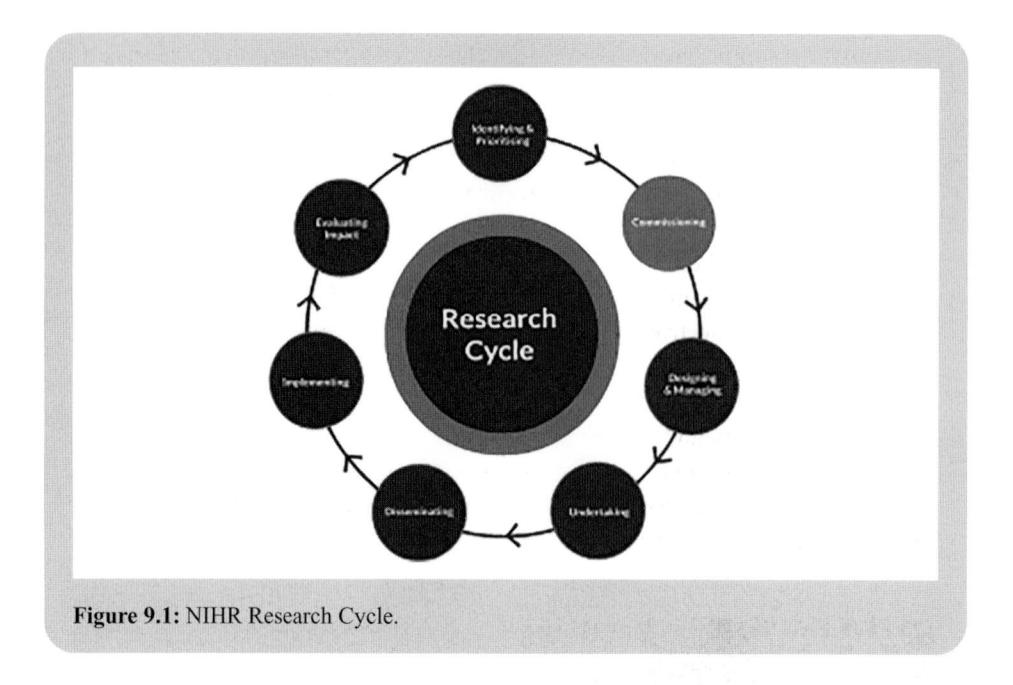

process. Smaller trusts which do not have this capacity are supported by local Clinical Research Networks (CRN).

There are also 10 NIHR Research Design Services[20] across England who help with research design, and identify suitable sources of funding - as well as involving patients and public in the research process.

Research in the NHS
Background
Research is core to the NHS principle of maintaining the highest standards of excellence and professionalism:

> "..through its promotion, conduct and use (of research) to improve the current and future health and care of the population" NHS Constitution.

Clinical research in the NHS means undertaking studies which generate 'evidence' to inform health professionals about what they need to do to improve care, e.g. by determining which healthcare intervention or treatments work best.

Healthcare professionals undertake many roles in clinical research, e.g. leading research, recruiting participants, and promoting participation in research by patients and the public. Furthermore, evidence suggests 'research-active NHS' hospitals have better patient care outcomes.

New treatments researched may include new drugs, different surgical techniques, or novel medical devices. For example, open surgery may be replaced with a non-surgical intervention

---
20. Yes, another silo!

such as a radiological technique or enhanced physiotherapy. Also, without evidence from research, there is the risk patients are given treatments that provide no benefit or are detrimental.

Aim of Clinical Research

Clinical research aims to find out if new treatments:
- Are safe
- Have any side effects
- Provide better patient outcomes than the current standard of care
- Are more cost effective than the current standard of care.

Examples of Clinical Research

Examples of clinical research include testing:
- Vaccines to prevent the spread of an illness or a virus, e.g. C19
- New scans or imaging techniques enabling more accurate diagnoses
- Less invasive tests instead of invasive clinical procedures

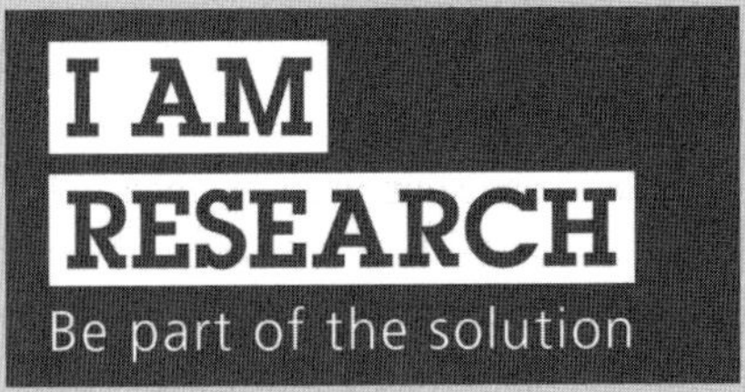

Figure 9.2: You can be part of the solution.

Research	Service Evaluation	Clinical Audit
Derive new knowledge	Define or judge current care	Inform delivery of best care
Test hypothesis / explore themes	What standard does this service achieve?	Does this service achieve a predetermined standard?
Define questions, aims and objectives	Measures without reference to a standard	Measures against a standard
New / routine treatment, sample or investigation data	Analysis of existing data	Analysis of existing data
May involve allocating patients to interventions	Intervention chosen before evaluation	Intervention chosen before audit
May involve randomisation	No randomisation	No randomisation
Will require ethical approval	No HRA or ethical approval	No HRA or ethical approval

Figure 9.3: Differences between Research, Service Evaluation and Clinical Audit.

- New drugs or medical devices
- Other healthcare interventions that control a patient's illness or improve their quality of life, e.g. researching whether a particular diet affects a condition, or further preparing patients for surgery by improving their fitness.

Clinical Research is often confused with Clinical Audit or Service Evaluation. In a healthcare setting, the generation of *new* knowledge defines whether the activity is research. There are also other differences highlighted in Figure 9.3.

Types of Research Studies

Qualitative and Quantitative Research

Clinical research can be qualitative, quantitative or both. Qualitative research can be divided into:
- Case study
- Narrative
- Ethnography (drawn from anthropology)
- Phenomenological (drawn from philosophy)
- 'Grounded theory' (drawn from sociology).

Qualitative research methods mainly involve interview or observation or both.

Quantitative research is of two types: observational studies and intervention studies (often called trials). Observational studies can be descriptive and/or analytical. Their main types are Cross-sectional studies, Cohort studies, Case-control studies, Ecological studies and Case series. Critically, all intervention studies are analytical in nature. They are further divided into randomised control trials and non-randomised control trials.

A combination of qualitative and quantitative techniques can often be used

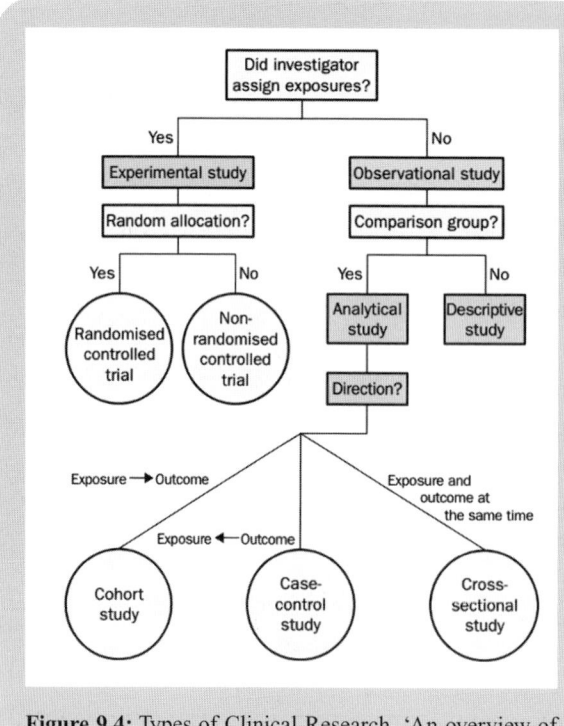

Figure 9.4: Types of Clinical Research. 'An overview of clinical research: the lay of the land'.

and is known as 'mixed-methods research'. The range of clinical research is summarised in Figure 9.4.

Sampling and Randomisation
Research cannot be done in a whole population due to insurmountable constraints such as funding, time, and resources. Instead, it is standard practice to take a smaller *sample* population.

Sampling in qualitative research includes judgement (purposive), accessibility (convenience), quota or haphazard sampling. Conversely, in quantitative research a random sample (see Figure 9.5) is the gold standard for sampling; depending on the nature of what is being researched, randomisation can be simple or complex.

Methodology
A core part of research is to describe the method to be used (methodology). This includes study type, outcomes to be included/measured, sampling methods, determining sample size and statistical analysis.

Before starting quantitative research, it is necessary to consult a medical statistician to calculate sample size. Also, with their advice, one can decide on the statistical method to be used, to analyse the data. An epidemiologist may also be needed to help design the research.

Research Ideas
All research studies start with an idea. This usually centres on how current clinical practice can be improved. These ideas can come from:
- Observing current practice
- Speaking to patients and/or care providers to obtain their opinions
- Finding out what improvements have been tested elsewhere and asking if the new idea can work in a clinical setting.

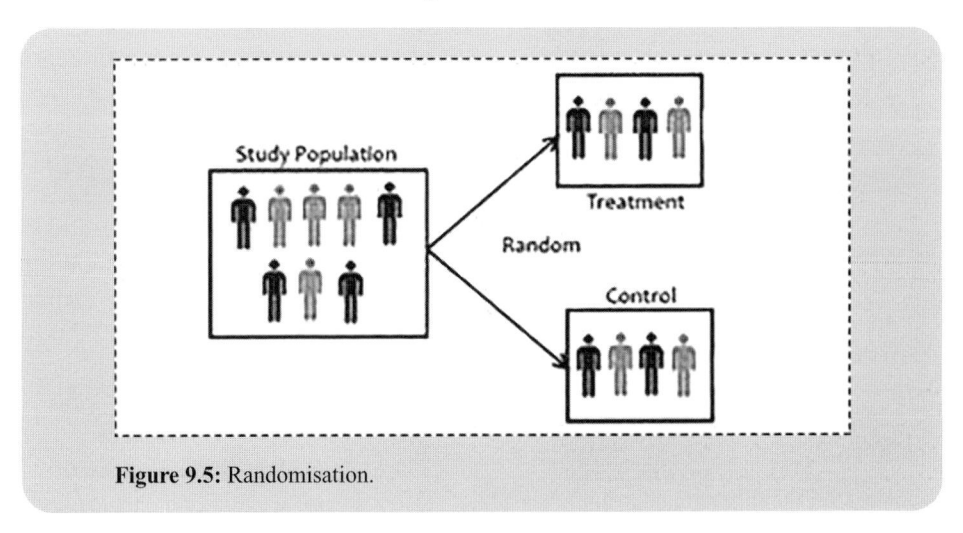

Figure 9.5: Randomisation.

Generating Ideas via Clinical Audit or Service Evaluation
Both service improvement and audit can lead to the generation of research ideas. A clinical audit which measures outcome (against a well-defined standard of practice) may identify changes needed. This can generate research ideas to test whether these changes are effective. Similarly, a service evaluation that assesses what a clinical service is achieving (for example against accepted performance indicators) may generate research ideas.

Generating Ideas from Previous Research
One of the most common ways of generating a research idea is from the analysis of previous research. This can involve looking at studies that have been undertaken in other countries, hospitals or certain patient populations; and predicting their impact in your local population. Alternatively, it may involve the same study being repeated some years later, to validate or refute the previous results.

Developing Research Questions
The next step is to turn a research idea into a research question. A research question needs to be clear, focused, concise and arguable. It also needs to be:
- Important - it must be a question that needs to be answered
- New - it must never have been answered in a clinical environment, or novel in terms of needing to be answered in a *different* clinical environment
- Clear and specific - so that the answer is also clear and specific
- Relevant - to the NHS and to patients.

'PICO' (which stands for Population, Intervention, Comparison and Outcome) is a widely used strategy for framing research questions. It is used to clarify the research question and determine the type of study most appropriate to answer the question, see Figure 9.6.

P	I	C	O
Population Patient Problem	Intervention or Exposure	Comparison	Outcome
Who are the patients? What is the problem?	What do we do to them? What are they exposed to?	What do we compare the intervention with?	What happens? What is the outcome?

Figure 9.6: The PICO Model.

Consider the following research question: 'does robotic surgery lead to a better clinical outcome compared to conventional surgery?'. After determining this question, the PICO approach is followed:

- **P**   Patients requiring surgery
- **I**   Robotic surgery
- **C**   *vs* Conventional surgery
- **O**   Better clinical outcomes.

A common challenge facing researchers is deciding how best to present a research question, so it engages those reading or reviewing the study.

Research Funding

Why Research Funding is Needed
Research activity is not classed as primarily 'patient care', and therefore is not funded through normal NHS commissioning (purchasing) routes. To ensure research can be undertaken without being a burden on NHS resources, external funding is required.

The main types of costs associated with research studies include:
- Staff time - investigators, research staff and technicians, statisticians, and research management, governance, administration, etc.
- Other costs - equipment, consumables, travel expenses, conferences, etc.

It is important to understand the distinction between the cost of research and the funding obtained:
- Cost   = how much it will cost the NHS to undertake the research
- Funding = how much the NHS requests (or receives) from the funder.

In many cases, funders will only fund the *direct* costs of the research and not the *indirect* costs, e.g. overheads. The Full Economic Costs (FECs) of research studies include both direct and indirect costs.

Research Funders
Figure 9.7 gives an overview of some of the main funders of clinical research in the UK and their schemes, with an indication of how much funding is available. Grant funders may be specifically focused on one health specialty (e.g. oncology), or will be more general. In addition, depending on size and complexity, different funders will be more applicable for different studies.

Many R&D departments within NHS hospitals have funding experts who provide further advice and information on funders and their programmes. They can also help researchers prepare and cost funding applications.

Funder	Main Programmes	Funding Limit	What will be funded
National Institute of Health Research	Efficacy and Mechanism Evaluation Health Services and Delivery Research Health Technology Assessment Programme Grants for Applied Research Research for Patient Benefit	Varies from around £50,000 to over £1 million depending on the programme	100% NHS direct costs 80% FEC for higher education institutions
UK Research & Innovation	EPSRC plus Fellowships Innovate UK MRC plus Fellowships	Varies from around £50,000 to over £1 million	80% FEC 100% NHS directs costs plus overheads
Association of Medical Research Charities	British Heart Foundation Cancer Research UK Versus Arthritis Wellcome Trust	Varies from about £50,000 to over £1 million	100% of directly incurred costs, i.e. salaries that are dependent on the funding
Local Charities	Varies depending on geographical location	Up to £25,000	Up to 100% of direct costs
Commercial / Industry Funders	Pharmaceutical and other healthcare companies	Varies for different industry funders	Full economic cost (direct and indirect costs)

Figure 9.7: Some of the Major Funders of Clinical Research in the UK.

Preparing Grant Applications

Research funding applications will vary for different funders. But, in general, all require the following information:

- **Background** - to the research, similar to a literature review. This should highlight gaps in the current research and make the case for the research
- **Research plan** - with clear aims and objectives, that is scientifically sound, realistic, and with defined outcomes or outputs
- **Study design and methodology** - to answer the research question, including a description of the sample size, data collection methods and approach to analysis

- **Skills and expertise** - of the research team, which will depend on the complexity and size of the research
- **Dissemination and impact** - of the results. This should not only include publications or conferences attended, but also demonstrate the benefits to patients and the NHS
- **Management of funders** - who will expect to see an explanation of how the research will be achieved on time and within budget
- **Cost of the research** - and funding requested as per the funder's criteria.

Characteristics of a Good Grant Application
The following are important when preparing good quality applications:
- **Clearly written sections** - that help the reviewer grasp your study, understand the importance of your research question, and how your methodology will answer it. This can be achieved by:
    - Using headings, sub-headings and paragraphs
    - **Bolding** important text so it stands out
    - Using plain English, explaining abbreviations and avoiding jargon
    - Using diagrams or flow charts to demonstrate how patients will be involved in the study, or to explain complex procedures.
- **Correct grammar and spellings** - and proofread carefully
- **Patient public involvement** - funding applications are greatly improved by patient perspectives. Active Patient and Public Involvement (PPI) is a requirement for most grant funders. This leads to the important NIHR research principle:

".. research (*should be*) carried out 'with' or 'by' members of the public rather than 'to', 'about' or 'for' them".

Research Costs
Research studies should be costed accurately and offer value for money. They also need to meet eligibility criteria, which will vary depending on the funder. The funding rules regarding costs can be complicated. Research studies that take place within the NHS additionally need to consider:
- **Research costs** - associated with core research activities being undertaken to answer the research questions. These costs end when the research ends. These costs are usually met by grant funders
- **Treatment costs** - associated with patient care activities integral to the provision of a treatment. These costs will continue after the research. These costs are met through the normal NHS service
- **Service support costs** - associated with patient care activities not integral to the provision of a treatment (and that will end when the research ends). These costs are met from the R&D budget of the health departments in the UK.

This breakdown of costs is in line with DH's 'Attributing the costs of health and social care Research and Development' (AcoRD) guidance. This provides a framework to identify, recover and attribute NHS costs. Accurate attribution of the costs of research studies can be complex. It is therefore advisable support is obtained from AcoRD specialists in R&D departments in NHS hospitals, or the CRN.

Top Tips (to obtain funding)
- Funding can help to pay for staff time thereby releasing staff from their clinical duties
- Well-written and accurately costed grant applications will increase the chance of studies receiving funding
- Support from R&D departments and regional organisations can help with preparing competitive funding applications.

Further Support
In addition to support provided by R&D departments, further support can be obtained from the funders themselves or the following regional bodies.

Clinical Research Networks (CRNs)
CRNs support patients, the public and health and care organisations across England to participate in high-quality research. The 'early contact teams' in different regions can provide advice on funding applications.

Research Design Service (RDS)
An RDS provides support for researchers preparing peer-reviewed grant applications. This includes support for research design, research methods, statistics, health economics and involving patients. Some regional RDSs provide a small amount of funding for PPI activities to inform larger grant funding applications.

Principles and Starting

Research Governance and Ethics
Research Ethics are considerations that must be made throughout the life cycle of a research project – from concept, right the way through to publication and dissemination.

Research Governance (RG) ensures high standards in research, which includes ethics. RG includes regulations and checks before the research can begin.

At its heart, RG aims to safeguard patients, protect researchers and ensure good quality research, while mitigating risks. The UK Policy Framework for Health & Social Care Research (UKPFHSC) sets out RG principles including:
- **Ethics** - the dignity, rights, safety, and wellbeing of participants must be the primary consideration
- **Science** - ensure only high quality, valid research is conducted, as determined by independent reviews

- **Health & Safety** - research may use potentially dangerous equipment and substances; therefore ensuring the safety of patients and researchers is vital
- **Transparency** - ensure public access to information on research being conducted and its findings
- **Finance** - ensure financial probity; checking there is adequate insurance cover; and arrangements are in place regarding intellectual property
- **Quality** - promoting excellence in research in the UK.

Role of Sponsor and Chief Investigator (CI)

All research conducted in health and social care must have a sponsor. The UKPFHSC states that a sponsor is an:

> ".. individual, or organisation that takes on overall responsibility for proportionate, effective arrangements being in place to set up, run and report on a research project".

All studies also need a Chief Investigator, or 'CI'. They are the 'boss' of the study and take overall medicolegal responsibility for it.

Different Types of Approval

Typically, a study involving NHS patients, or healthy volunteers, requires the following regulatory approvals:
- HRA
- Research Ethics Committee (REC)
- Confirmation of Capacity and Capability (C&C).

If the project involves the use of medicinal products or devices, approval from the Medicines and Healthcare products Regulatory Agency (MHRA) will also be required.

Integrated Research Application System (IRAS) Form

Approvals must be requested through the Integrated Research Application System (IRAS), a single system designed to capture all the information required for a project. The IRAS form enables the applicant(s) to provide information once for all the various review bodies.

Carrying out Research
Start
Consent

Participant-informed consent forms the basis/principles of Good Clinical Practice (GCP) and is a basic human right. GCP defines consent as:

> "A process by which a subject voluntarily confirms his or her willingness to participate in a particular trial after having been informed of all aspects of the trial that are relevant to the subject's decision to participate. Informed consent is documented by means of a written, signed and dated informed consent form".

The Medicines for Human Use (Clinical Trials) Regulations (2004) also requires consent in clinical trials. A clinical trial requires freely given informed consent by all subjects as well as:
- Significant focus on the protection of participants (particularly vulnerable groups)
- Legal representation for vulnerable patients unable to give informed consent (including children)
- 'Prior interview' for informed consent
- A contact point for all trial subjects.

Randomisation and Blinding
The majority of clinical trials involve randomisation. This is the process by which participants are allocated to an arm of trial in a random manner. Randomisation is important as it minimises selection bias, preventing the emergence of misleading findings. This is achieved by allocation concealment, whereby researchers do not know (and cannot guess), what the next participant's treatment allocation will be.

Randomisation also balances the participants in each trial arm for both known and unknown confounding variables. This means any differences between the arms will be due to chance, and any differences in outcome measures can be attributed to the treatment allocated.

Random allocation is usually determined by a computer programme or can be pre-written on a Master Randomisation List by a statistician.

Blinding is another important element of clinical trials which minimises bias. It means the participant or outcome assessor alone (single blinding), or both (double blinding), do not know what treatment is being administered post-randomisation.

Middle
Data Collection at Various Time Points
High quality data is imperative to high quality research. The time points for the data required will be set out by the protocol. This data may take many forms, e.g. a blood result, biomedical variable (blood pressure or weight), x-rays, or a health questionnaire.

Intervention vs Standard Care
Many research studies compare standard care (i.e. what NHS patients would usually get), with another intervention, to determine which leads to better outcomes. In these studies, participants will be randomised to either the standard care ('control') arm or the intervention ('treatment') arm.

In terms of data collection, the activities during the trial should be the same for both sets of participants, except for their standard care or the intervention. In essence, both arms are designed to appear identical to 'blinded' participants/investigators. Some research studies involve many NHS sites and hence standard care may differ between these sites; therefore, to ensure validity, the protocol needs to define what constitutes standard care.

Data Analysis
Data analysis happens at varying time points depending on the type of study. Sometimes an interim analysis is required to ensure the research is gaining enough data; or it may only happen at the end of the study once all data is collected. Researchers will use different statistical software systems depending on the type of data to be analysed.

Monitoring/Governance
The purpose of monitoring a research study is to ensure the practices being performed are in keeping with the study protocol.

End
Close Down
According to the HRA:

> "The definition of the end of study is detailed in the protocol as being the date of the last visit of the last participant or the completion of follow up monitoring and data collection".

Closing involves ending the study in all sites, and/or declaring the end of a study. Closedown is a time where all documentation can be finalised, and all costs completed. The absolute end of a study is when research findings are shared with all participating sites, and the results are in the process of being published. This must include those which don't support the initial hypothesis (i.e. negative findings).

Publication
Good clinical research needs to be shared with colleagues, participants, and the national and international healthcare community. This is done in various ways:
- Writing to participants
- Presentations to colleagues
- Presentations at conferences
- Publishing scientific papers in the 'highest impact' (i.e. most important) journal possible.

Trial Management Unit (TMU)
A TMU is especially useful to help manage NHS research which is complex and time consuming. Trial management is vital for the successful delivery of any research study, as it will make sure the project meets its recruitment target on time, and within budget. Importantly, trial management staff also ensure the research study is being conducted according to GCP. This is essential for maintaining patient safety and data integrity.

The UK Trial Managers' Network provides useful resources, as well as providing support for those carrying out trial management activities. In some larger NHS hospitals, there is an 'in house' TMU which helps deliver research. Here are some examples of how a TMU can help.

Protocol Design
A TMU can help develop the protocol and act as a central point of contact between the sponsor, funder, and investigators.

Randomisation
TMU staff will work with statisticians and the CI to decide upon the most appropriate randomisation procedure for the clinical trial; as well as hosting access to an emergency unblinding procedure (to reveal a participant's random allocation in an emergency).

Integrated Research Approval System Application
A TMU will support investigators to complete IRAS forms and to apply for appropriate regulatory and ethical approval.

Amendments
If any documentation (or procedure) is changed following initial approval, these will need to be approved prior to use. This does not apply to urgent safety measures which should be implemented immediately by the research staff, and then followed by the submission of an amendment. The study sponsor, site R&D department, and TMU staff support researchers who need to submit an amendment for their study.

Administration
A TMU will arrange regular meetings which are important for the successful delivery of a trial. Additionally, it will help collate the appropriate information required to monitor the trial, ensuring it is delivered as per protocol and GCP guidelines.

Site Set-up and Coordination
A TMU will help identify other sites that could participate in the trial by contacting the CRNs and R&D departments in different NHS trusts. Furthermore, once the sites are located, a TMU will support the site set-up procedures.

Data Management
Data management ensures data collected is complete and accurately entered onto the trial database ready for statistical analysis. A Data Management Plan (DMP) is usually written at the start of a trial and outlines how the data will be collected and corrected if required.

Archiving and Close Down
Following the resolution of queries and the 'study close-out' by the CI, all essential trial documentation will usually be transferred to a third-party archiving service (which should provide suitable fire and water-resistant facilities).

The TMU will support this procedure, ensuring the relevant trial documents and data are archived for the necessary time (usually 15 years).

Research

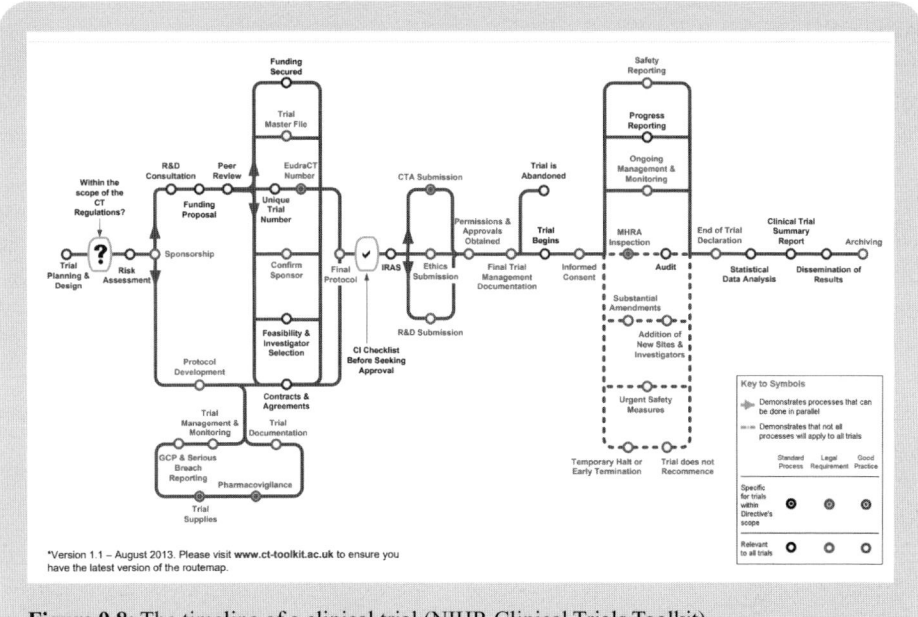

Figure 9.8: The timeline of a clinical trial (NIHR Clinical Trials Toolkit).

Summary
There is a lot to do when a research study is planned and performed. This is summarised in the (rather complex) Figure 9.8, which is copied from the NIHR Clinical Trials Toolkit. A TMU can help a lot. The route map goes through the main timeline of a Clinical Trial (designed in the style of the London Underground Tube Map). Users can click on each 'station' to get more detailed advice and information at each stage.

Patient and Public Involvement (PPI)
PPI is necessary to get funding and to publish research studies. PPI refers to members of the public being actively involved in research projects and research organisations. PPI is distinctly different to people taking part in research as research participants.

Members of the public, including patients and carers, offer alternative and valuable perspectives to research, especially in areas in which they have life-experience. This could include living with a particular condition, caring for or living with someone with this condition, or being within a certain demographic group. PPI can result in higher quality and more relevant research being designed and undertaken. This is recognised by organisations, such as the NIHR and HRA, who assess how the public have been involved in the research when applications are reviewed.

It is important researchers plan, prepare, and implement PPI in their research as early as possible; considering how they wish to involve people, and who they would like to involve. The UK Standards for Public Involvement are designed to improve the quality and consistency of public involvement in research.

Research Impact

It is not enough to publish your results. 'Research impact' is the true value of clinical research. All clinical research sets out with a hypothesis and objectives, but due to the nature of conducting research in a clinical setting, these are not always realised. However, research results can lead to substantial changes in clinical care and treatment pathways. Here are some examples:

Example 1 – Autosomal Dominant Polycystic Kidney Disease

Autosomal Dominant Polycystic Kidney Disease (ADPKD) is an inherited cause of kidney failure. Dialysis may be required in the later stages, and there is no specific treatment for the underlying disease. A large worldwide multicentre study was conducted over 10 years, including at the author's hospital, concerning a drug treatment named 'Tolvaptan' which is now part of a NICE guideline on ADPKD.

The hospital now runs monthly Tolvaptan clinics and offers a treatment for a disease that previously had no treatment option.

Example 2 – COVID-19

More recently the impact and translation of clinical research into clinical practice has been seen with the C19 pandemic. The largest UK clinical trial in 2020, looking at treatment options for this new disease - called the 'RECOVERY Trial' – ran across multiple sites, in a bid to gain an understanding of the disease and of what treatments would be effective.

Global interest initially centred around the impact of Hydroxychloroquine on acutely unwell C19 patients. However this treatment was shown not to be effective. It did however find Dexamethasone (a low-cost steroid) was effective, and this was adopted clinically via a rapid NICE guideline. The study continues to review and influence practice by examining anti-rheumatic drugs, antibodies and anti-inflammatories. By the time you are reading this, the list will have expanded again.

Example 3 – Leg Fractures

Another study (on open leg fractures) has been conducted at the author's hospital, along with 23 other UK hospitals. It demonstrated there is no difference in patient recovery between high-tech negative pressure 'wound therapy devices' and standard dressings.

Summary

Conducting healthcare research has evolved over the years and has become a separate entity, with cutting-edge scientific research being conducted throughout the NHS. Such research often requires a team of multi-specialty experts comprising clinicians, public health workers, epidemiologists, medical statisticians, R&D and TMU teams - and members of the public.

Research is the future of patient care and service improvement. Without it, the NHS cannot sustain, or improve, the care we provide.

Further reading

The Lancet. Epidemiology of research design useful papers.

https://www.thelancet.com/series/epidemiology

https://www.thelancet.com/series/epidemiology-2002

The NIHR. Clinical Research Networks.

https://www.nihr.ac.uk/explore-nihr/support/clinical-research-network.htm

Royal College of Physicians. Recognising research: how research improves patient care.

https://www.rcplondon.ac.uk/news/recognising-research-how-research-improves-patient-care

Chapter 10

The Digital NHS

"The biggest part of our digital transformation is changing the way we think."
Simeon Preston, BUPA.

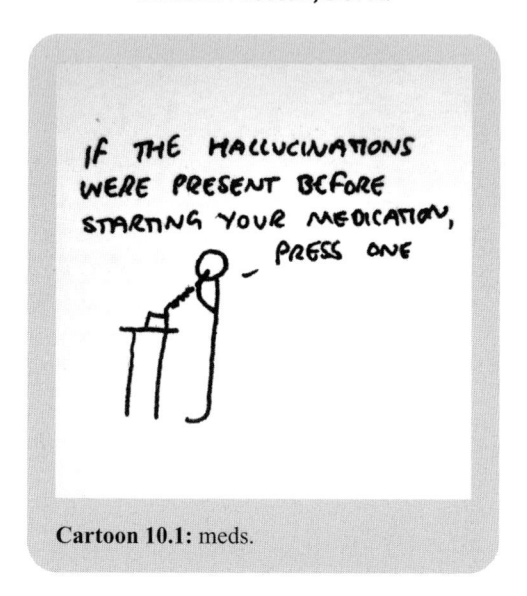

> IF THE HALLUCINATIONS WERE PRESENT BEFORE STARTING YOUR MEDICATION, PRESS ONE

Cartoon 10.1: meds.

Introduction

This quote is as true for healthcare as for any part of society. The NHS has progressed immensely over its 70 plus years, but the development of healthcare computer technology has often lagged behind.

There are two contrasting aspects to the 'digital NHS'. Firstly, innovative digital infrastructure enables patients and healthcare providers (us!) to benefit greatly from intuitive and reliable resources. But secondly, countless outdated and incongruent digital systems further burden the NHS, making the organisation much less efficient.

Each day in the NHS:
- £57,534 is saved through automated electronic services (a saving which increases each year)
- 500,000 NHS professionals access applications hosted by NHS Digital
- 750,000 electronic referrals are processed
- 2,000,000 electronic prescriptions are processed
- 302,400,000 secure, electronic messages are sent.

The Digital NHS

Primary care is a classic example of these two sides. Across the UK, GPs work from electronic patient records (EPRs)[21]. EPRs hold significant volumes of data, such as notes from consultations, blood tests, other investigations, and copies of correspondence from other healthcare providers. However, general practices hold EPRs on one of four systems: TPP SystmOne, EMIS web, InPS Vision, and Microtest Evolution - which do not necessarily 'talk to' each other. Furthermore, general practices are emailed (and sent paper letters) from different hospitals and must spend time transferring them into their systems.

There are systems in place where primary care and other aspects of the NHS have integrated successfully, e.g. when a GP prescribes a medication, the patient can now select their preferred pharmacy. Their medication is then prepared at the dispensing pharmacy before the patient leaves the practice. Since the 1980s, general practices have used technology to reduce workload, such as through computerised repeat prescribing. But secondary care has been slow to follow.

Nonetheless some advances have been made in secondary care. An example is the Picture Archiving and Communication System (PACS) which allows healthcare professionals to access (past and present) x-ray, CT, MRI, and US images, at any healthcare centre with PACS. One benefit of this, for example, is that a CT head taken at 4am in the UK can be interpreted in a southern hemisphere country like Australia (where it is daytime).

Despite such advances, the 'digital NHS' is 'patchy', partly because of technology historically being 'out-sourced'; with long-term, overlapping contracts from private companies preventing NHS organisations from modernising effectively.

Digital NHS Landscape – Evolution and Current State

When considering the use of technology in the NHS, it is vital to consider how its use has developed in primary and secondary care, and at national level. Figure 10.2 shows a timeline for the development of digital in the NHS.

Spine I was a programme developed to serve as the backbone of a national IT infrastructure. The DH formed the 'NHS Connecting for Health (CfH) Agency' in March 2005 out of the NHS Information Authority, to develop a national NHS IT Infrastructure.

Spine I had multiple services feeding in, such as electronic prescribing, electronic appointments booking, integrated care records, PACS and a central email directory. It had

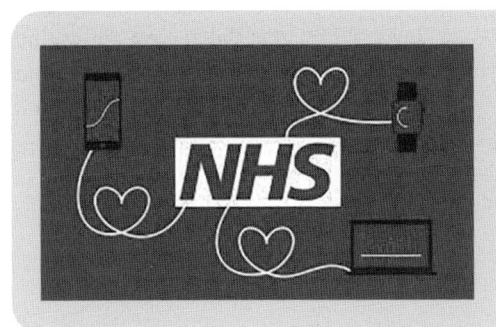

Figure 10.1: The Digital NHS logo.

---

21. Yup, another acronym-positive chapter!

	Primary Care	**Secondary Care**	**Governmental/NHS Management**
1965-1970	The first use of computers in general practice (Dr John Preece, Exeter)	The first use of ward computers to access clinical test results	
1975	The first paperless general practice (Ottery St Mary Health Centre)		
1990s	Up to 96% general practices have computers, 15% now paperless (1996)	Introduction of Picture Archiving and Communications System (PACS)	Personal Child Health Record introduced into NHS structure (1991)
2001		First robotic surgery performed, St Mary's London	
2003		76% consultants have NHSnet email and browsing access	NHSnet (NHSmail and browser services) launched through British Telecom (BT)
2004			NHS Integrated Care Records Services launched
2005	Choose and Book online service launched		Health & Social Care Information Centre (HSCIC) launched, Connecting for Health (CfH) agency formed, Spine I launched, NHS Electronic Prescription Service
2006			New National Network (N3) formed
2010		Lorenzo adopted to the first hospital, providing electronic patient record platform	
2013			NHSmail2 launched, NHS Digital launched
2014			Spine II launched
2017	GP at Hand/ Babylon GP launched in London		NHS Identity Service (Health and Social Care Network – HSCN) – replaced N3
2018			NHS App launched (later useful for C19 Vaccination proof)
2019			NHSX formation
2021			NHS COVID-19 App used for contact tracing

Figure 10.2: Timeline of the development of NHS digital.

> PDS: This service hosts the demographic data relating to patients, stored under their NHS number. Whilst patients could not opt-out of this component of the Spine, they could request their personal data (such as name, contact details etc.) was hidden from healthcare staff.
>
> SCR: This service provides a summary of each patient's clinical details, including their health conditions, medications, and allergies.
>
> SUS: This service uses data from the PDS to support public health research, planning and delivery.

Figure 10.3: Spine 1 components.

three core components: Personal Demographics Service (PDS), Summary Care Record (SCR) and Secondary Uses Service (SUS).

At the start of 2007, 6.5 million records were hosted on the PDS, with 1.4 million patients using electronic booking services, and half a million uses of the electronic prescriptions service. Unfortunately, queries relating to the security of data and access to the Spine I system led to negative national press. In August 2014, as part of an effort to regain momentum by creating a centralised national IT infrastructure, Spine I was migrated to Spine II.

Spine II – the Current System in Operation

NHS Digital, working collaboratively with private technology firms, has built Spine II based on 12 Open-Source products – free platforms and services. Spine II includes systems to automate processes, reducing the need for costly maintenance and human resource administration.

Spine II is being developed to integrate and connect over 28,000 healthcare IT systems across 21,000 health and social care organisations. For example, paramedics across the UK may access SCRs for their patients remotely.

Over 65 million SCRs are available through Spine II. Spine II also hosts 90 million demographic records, sends 750,000 e-referral messages and over 2 million electronic prescriptions daily. The breadth of the Spine II infrastructure means over 500,000 NHS healthcare professionals access its hosted services each day. These include GPs making e-referrals, pharmacists checking medications and paramedics accessing SCRs - supporting more transactions daily than the UK's debit and credit card system.

NHS Identity – a Healthcare Staff Identity System

With the increasing demand and reliance on digital systems, healthcare professionals are provided with access to national systems through the Health and Social Care Network (HSCN). 'NHS Identity' can be considered the 'entry gatekeeper' to a significant volume of local NHS systems and associated data - meaning this (one) system must be robust, reliable and secure.

The HSCN replaced something called N3 in April 2017 and uses multifactor authentication to provide access to NHS systems. These authentications use NHS Smartcards, pin codes or biometrics (e.g. fingerprint/facial recognition). Whilst NHS Digital is currently delivering this service at the local trust level, the longer-term goal is to create a single national system of access to NHS Identity, which allows staff (and patients) access to systems.

NHS Net/NHS Mail

The NHS needs reliable, clear, immediate, effective and secure communication across teams, departments and Trusts. Historically, facsimile (fax) machines were used, providing a very secure method of transferring documentation and correspondence. Whilst the use of fax machines is outdated – the Secretary of State for Health declared their phasing out in 2018 – they are still in use in the NHS.

NHSmail2 – the current NHS email system – has protection from inappropriate access, but there are errors caused by users and the ability to identify emails within the NHSmail2 system. In November 2016, one NHS staff member emailed approximately 850,000 others a 'test' email, after a bug in the NHSmail2 system included everyone in an email distribution list. The issue was conflated by the 'reply all' function. This led to approximately 500 million emails sent across the system in 75 minutes, causing delays and disruption.

That said, the predominant communication method is now secure email, through NHSmail2. NHSmail2 includes measures that protect against the loss of information and inappropriate access, using advanced encryption technologies. If communicating with non-secure email addresses, writing '[secure]' at the start of the subject line will encrypt the correspondence. The recipient then needs to register to access the file, which opens the email in a secure window on an internet browser.

NHS Digital and the NHS App

The Health and Social Care Information Centre (HSCIC) was created by a merger of parts of the NHS Information Authority, and the Prescribing Support Unit. Following the Health and Social Care Act 2012, the HSCIC changed from a 'special health authority' to an 'executive non-departmental public body'. HSCIC then took over parts of the troubled NHS National Programme for IT from the NHS CfH agency (which ceased to exist). It also runs the Health Survey for England. In July 2016, HSCIC was rebranded 'NHS Digital'.

NHS Digital has oversight of the NHS Apps Library, the NHS Website, NHS 111 website, and the NHS A-Z directory. As part of NHS Digital's aim to increase access to healthcare services and information, they launched the NHS App in January 2019.

For patients to use the NHS App, the NHS needs to ensure the identity of the person following a strict process. Initially, details such as full name, date of birth, contact details and unique NHS Number are required. Then, after confirming contact details, the app requires photographic evidence of accepted ID forms, such as a passport or driving licence. The app then requires a photo or video from the mobile phone

> **The NHS App (launched Jan 2019)** has several invaluable services built in:
>
> - **Book appointments electronically** – patients can search for, book and manage appointments at their GP surgery.
> - **View personal medical records** – patients can securely access your GP records and see information such as allergies, and current/past medications.
> - **Register/de-register for organ donation** – patients can provide information about their decisions regarding organ donation.
> - **Review how the NHS uses personal data** – patients can choose how their health records are shared for research and planning.
> - **Message healthcare professionals or submit online forms for clinical review** – patients may be sent, and can return, information or templated forms to complete as part of their consultation.
> - **Access health services on behalf of someone you care for** – this app is also available for appropriate access by carers for individuals who may have complex healthcare needs.

Figure 10.4: The components of the NHS App.

of the person registering, to verify the face of the person registering against the ID submitted. Following verification of information submitted (which takes approximately two hours), access to the NHS App's full list of functions is granted. Have a go. It is very good.

Picture Archiving and Communication System – a Radiological Breakthrough

PACS is a Spine I success story and is designed to be a single point of access to radiological images. This system has four fundamental uses:

1. **Radiology workflow management** - radiologists use it to structure their daily patient workflow, reviewing and reporting radiological information
2. **Electronic image hosting** - decreasing the physical limitations of storage
3. **Remote access to medical imaging** - allowing clinicians to access medical images without being present at a specific Trust. This allows for international collaborations, distanced reporting and training; and for multiple healthcare professionals to access the image at the same time
4. **Image integration** - images can be integrated with other clinical electronic systems.

PACS is constantly developing, with input from both radiologists and other clinical sectors, such as clinical laboratories, oncology, cardiology, etc. PACS is an incredibly rich data source but must comply with strict regulations. Automated processes are built into PACS when images are archived, ensuring patient details associated with the images

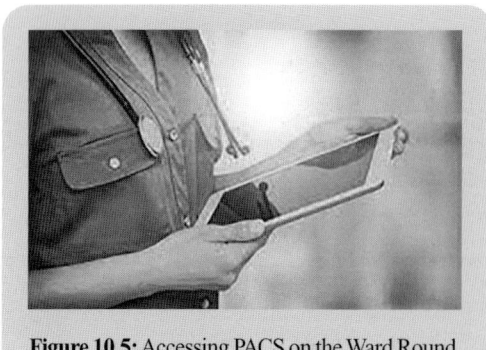

Figure 10.5: Accessing PACS on the Ward Round.

are correct. Images are archived and stored using a platform called DICOM (Digital Imaging and Communications in Medicine). PACS and DICOM have revolutionised the quality and effectiveness of radiology throughout the NHS.

Among the images PACS holds are those from: ultrasounds, MRI scans, x-rays, endoscopies, mammograms and histopathology.

Digital NHS: From Cradle to Grave
To understand the different systems currently used in the NHS, we will follow the life of a typical patient. One thing to keep in mind whilst reading this section, is that these systems were developed independently. And whilst they may feed into one another, significant amounts of data still flow between services using (incomplete) paper-based methods.

NHSX, Midwifery and Maternity Services
In April 2019, the DHSC set up NHSX incorporating NHS Digital, NHS Improvement, NHS England and countless local services. NHSX aims to drive digital, data and technological reform throughout health and social care, including the development of 'Digital Maternity'.

When a child is born, a healthcare professional will register the birth on a local system, which automatically populates a message to the Personal Demographic Service (PDS) to notify them of the birth, and to assign the child their NHS Number. At this point, PDS informs the Child Health Record Department (CHRD) and registers the new-born on the Child Health Information System (CHIS).

CHIS automatically assigns the child a health visitor, and aids with scheduling a health visitor visit within 14 days. At 6-8 weeks following birth, CHIS automatically notifies parents to register the child with a local GP (and in turn, begin the Summary Care Record for that child), and attend a new-born health review. From this point forwards, the child then filters into the Healthy Children programme, which we outline later.

'Digital Maternity' will not only provide clear, concise, unbiased information to new mothers. It will also help healthcare staff, such as midwives and paediatricians, pass on key clinical information to health visitors and GPs - once mother and baby return home. NHSX's aim for 2023/2024 is that all women in the UK will have access to their maternity notes and information through their smart devices.

Child Health
In 2016 NHS England published the Healthy Children: Transforming Child Health guidance outlining current data and infrastructure in child health (Figure 1) - including

The Digital NHS

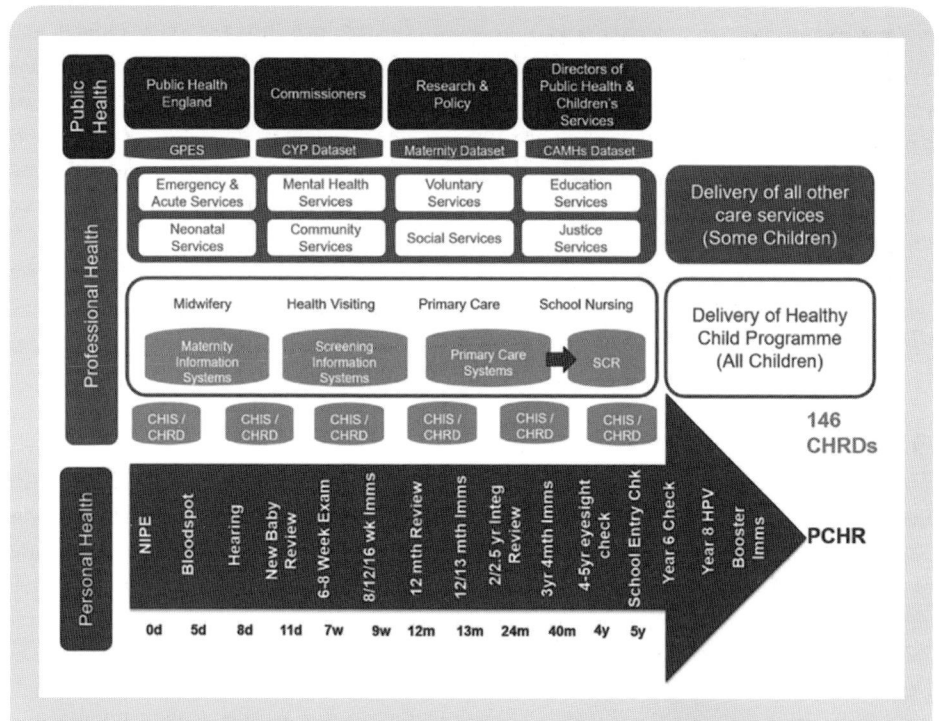

Figure 10.6: Public, professional and personal health pathways found within Children's Health in the UK, as described by NHS England in Healthy Children: Transforming Child Health.

aims for future developments. There are significant complexities around the provision of child health, and gaps in the current Child Health IT infrastructure.

The Personal Child Health Record (PCHR) is paper based. If lost, or not brought to clinical encounters, this means critical information may be assumed, missed or misremembered. The PCHR cannot be accessed remotely, meaning access to this information and auditing has become inordinately complex.

The CHIS may record Child Protection status and some ED attendances. However, as few care professionals have access to CHIS, useful information may be hidden. Overall, NHS England recognises that,

> "the current configuration of information services for children cannot guarantee knowing where a child is and how healthy they are, nor can they guarantee appropriate access to information for professionals".

End-of-Life Care

There are a few technological systems or devices available at the end-of-life such as 'electronic palliative care co-ordination systems'. They work 'behind the scenes' to enable multiple agencies to share the most up to date clinical information.

It is important patients can share their dying wishes and plan for a dignified death, e.g. they may possess a (written) 'Do Not Attempt Cardiopulmonary Resuscitation (DNACPR)' order; but if they are drowsy and an ambulance is called by someone not aware of this plan, they may be resuscitated against their will. Currently, the process of these wishes being documented is paper based, using a 'Red Form' (Recommended Summary Plan for Emergency Care and Treatment, ReSPECT) or other form of advance care planning.

When a person has died, a doctor must complete a paper medical death certificate. This must then be taken to the registrar for births, deaths and marriages. One day digital technology may help with the integration of death notification to relevant organisations (such as the NHS trusts and services the person has been using).

Currently, notification of the death of a patient to a GP is done by family members. Technology may in the future be able to revise the process, where a family member may notify the government (in a cyber-way) - through the registrar for births, deaths and marriages. An automated system could then identify the NHS organisations used by the deceased individual to update their systems. This should prevent, as sometime happens, automated communications to the deceased, which may distress relatives.

Ambulance Services

There are 14 autonomous Ambulance Trusts across the UK (10 in England), each with their own IT system (for example *GETAC* and *Siren*). Nonetheless paper has been (largely) removed from their patient record documentation. However, some ambulance services still use paper records concurrently to prevent data loss and for convenience.

One issue with the current BT-facilitated filter is that if someone calls emergency services from a different geographical location to the emergency, the caller automatically gets transferred to an Ambulance Trust unable to directly dispatch resources. So the first service needs to forward the call on to another service, delaying the dispatch of a paramedic.

As the 14 different Trusts work independently of each other - including triaging, managing emergency resource allocation, accessing pre-existing healthcare records and production of an electronic patient care record during that clinical episode - there is limited cohesion across systems. Also the 14 regions do not relate to the 7 NHSE regions – let alone the 13 HEE or 4 PHE regions. Blah blah blah.

For example, paramedics may attend someone with a lack of capacity and may not be able to access healthcare records because the patient is registered with a GP practice not registered to share details - or might only share partial data.

'NHS Pathways' is a triaging system used by some ambulance services. It directs approximately 19 million 111 and 999 triages each year. In the busiest month in 2020, August, this system triaged 1,660,085 calls (17.7% up from 2019); believed to be caused by the increased pressures of C19, and the perception of reduced access to primary healthcare.

1. When someone calls 999, this call is taken by a BT operative to filter to the emergency services
2. Using either the landline area code or nearby telephone mast the call is coming from, the call is automatically transferred to an emergency medical dispatcher for triaging
3. The triaging dispatcher follows protocols to assign triage code and allocate medical resources (ambulances, first responders etc). These either follow the NHS Pathways clinical tool or a private system called the Medical Priority Dispatch System (MPDS)
4. The emergency medical dispatcher continues to collect information and support the delivery of first aid information to the individual on the call, and sends patient identification details to the paramedics dispatched to the emergency
5. Paramedics may use the patient's date of birth, surname and address to identify their electronic primary care records, and access their past medical history, current medications, allergies, recent tests and consultations with their GP. Paramedics may also use the National Record Locator to find specific healthcare records such as mental health crisis plans, or the Medical Interoperability Gateway
6. Paramedics will create their own patient care record form for that patient, detailing the episode. Paramedics may also be able to access the patient's SCR through their tablet
7. Paramedics may use an audio video or call to nearby A&E departments for advice about how to prevent admission if appropriate. Paramedics can also notify the hospital about the incoming patient and relevant details to help the A&E department prepare for the patient's arrival
8. When the paramedics arrive at A&E, they handover to the A&E department. This is often verbal, transferring data collected on the electronic patient care reporting to the A&E department staff to document on their systems.

Figure 10.7: The process of calling an ambulance.

Primary Care Services, post-COVID-19

New technology-based services are now appearing in primary care. As well as the four systems for EPRs (and the innovative integration of these records into ambulance services), electronic prescribing is now linking better with pharmacy dispensers, and most secondary care referrals are electronic.

A commercial company, AccuRx, now provides a video-consultation service for the NHS (like an official 'NHS Microsoft Teams' or 'Zoom') to over 7,000 GP surgeries (and some hospitals) in the UK. AccuRx works across multiple electronic medical records systems, to provide GPs with SMS messaging to patients, patient triaging, photo sharing and video consultations. This technology may underpin most GP appointments in the future; and be an alternative to an appointment by telephone.

For example, during a telephone consultation, a patient may require healthcare support with a new skin complaint. The GP can send a SMS message to the patient's phone, providing a link to share images, and an information guide on how to take high-quality images. The images can then be reviewed by the GP, added to the patient's medical record, and shown to a consultant dermatologist - all done remotely.

Video consultations may also provide another depth to consultation; allowing the 'examination' of the area of the body where the complaint is centred. After consultations, GPs may also send approved resources and documents to help the patient understand their condition. During C19, AccuRx has been used by GPs as a primary method to ensure patients are being safely managed.

AccuRx, like other providers, has also developed a service to support C19 vaccination bookings; allowing availability of clinics to be shared, and monitor who has had the vaccine.

Secondary Care Services

Hospital IT Infrastructure is complex, predominantly because there are over 220 semi-independent hospital trusts in the UK, each organised and co-ordinated differently. The trusts work to deliver the DHSC's IT strategy, however the systems in place at each trust are ultimately locally chosen and may be bespoke or commercially sourced.

For example, in Yorkshire, a system called 'PPM+' was developed to create an 'electronic patient record (EPR)' initially to monitor cancer patients. PPM+ was then expanded into a trust-wide EPR system which can connect to EMIS (a common primary care patient record system); as well as PACS, local social care systems, national audits and numerous other trust-wide systems. PPM+ can also provide a platform for nursing staff to record observations, over-views of wards (referred to as 'eWhiteboards'), auto-populate handover documents, and trust-encrypted mobile devices.

Where PPM+ falls short, is it does not yet include data from all corners of healthcare provision; something that commercial providers (such as 'EPIC') are better equipped to provide. The ideal system would have all healthcare data included in an EPR for the whole of the NHS, and could be accessed via the NHS App, and NHS Identity.

The potential for use of intelligent technology in hospitals is vast. For example, minimally invasive surgery is being further developed using robotic surgery technology (called the 'daVinci Surgical System'). Telemedicine in theatres allows world-class surgeons to mentor operating surgeons and guide them through surgery. These two fields have been combined to support the delivery of remote surgery, with operations being performed with the surgeon in a different part of the world.

The Future of the Digital NHS
Distribution of Healthcare Resources

Over 2 billion people in the world lack access to vital medical services, such as blood tests, vaccination and emergency services. This includes countries facing economic and climate disruption such as Rwanda; where, for example, roads are often treacherous and (in monsoon season) impassable. To answer this issue, exciting developments in engineering have led to the creation of an 'autonomous drone delivery service' (called Zipline).

This technology has the possibility of supporting not only developing countries, but also during disaster relief and quarantine (when they could minimise human exposure to contagious diseases). Services mimicking Zipline may exist one day in the UK, improving accessibility to healthcare services and resources.

> A drone can be loaded with up to 1.6kg of medical stock and dispatched within 5 minutes. The drones rely on global positioning systems (GPS), which is fitted to the drone's battery. Novel technology within the drone identifies any obstacles and can alter the motor speed accordingly to prevent collision. These drones have a modular design, allowing for the rapid stocking, preparation of the drone on the launching system and ease of maintenance. The drone releases the resource safely from a hatch close to the ground, with the stock held in an insulated disposable cardboard box with connected parachute.

Figure 10.8: Drones.

Virtual Assistants in Healthcare (CERi)
The NHS works collaboratively with several external commercial companies to deliver its ambitious digital developments. With C19 causing unparalleled disruption to healthcare settings, NHS 111 saw an increase in demand of 257% in their online system in one year. Between June and November 2020, NHS111 online recorded 3,569,917 sessions – 860,213 of which specifically related to COVID-19.

In response, International Business Machines (IBM) worked with NHS 111 to develop an automated chatbot service to support patients who were requesting information regarding C19. This novel service, 'CERi' (Figure 10.9), incorporated state-of-the-art artificial intelligence (AI) search capability, to identify critical information from trusted sources regarding the virus. CERi was built to also display empathy to those using the service, and to evolve through user feedback.

'Syd' – See Yourself Differently
Current developments in the virtual assistant field aim to place health and well-being decisions into the pocket of the individual, as opposed to healthcare providers. Whilst there is a significant array of apps for calorie intake and exercise tracking, symptom monitoring, and medication compliance, few use artificial intelligence technology.

But one commercial application, 'Lamyiam', has created a personal smart health assistant called 'Syd'. Syd aims to provide a 'personalised health and well-being journey', through connecting the public with published research. The aim is to provide dynamic goals to help individuals build healthier lifestyles. This organisation collects lifestyle, genetic and personal data from their clients, creating tailored goals - and the assistant works to see how agreeable that is for the client.

However, this new market comes at a price. Not only is there the commercial cost of paying to access a virtual assistant, but data input such as genetic codes, shopping habits and exercise routines, is also required. Such data includes significant information about an individual, perhaps without appropriate regulation.

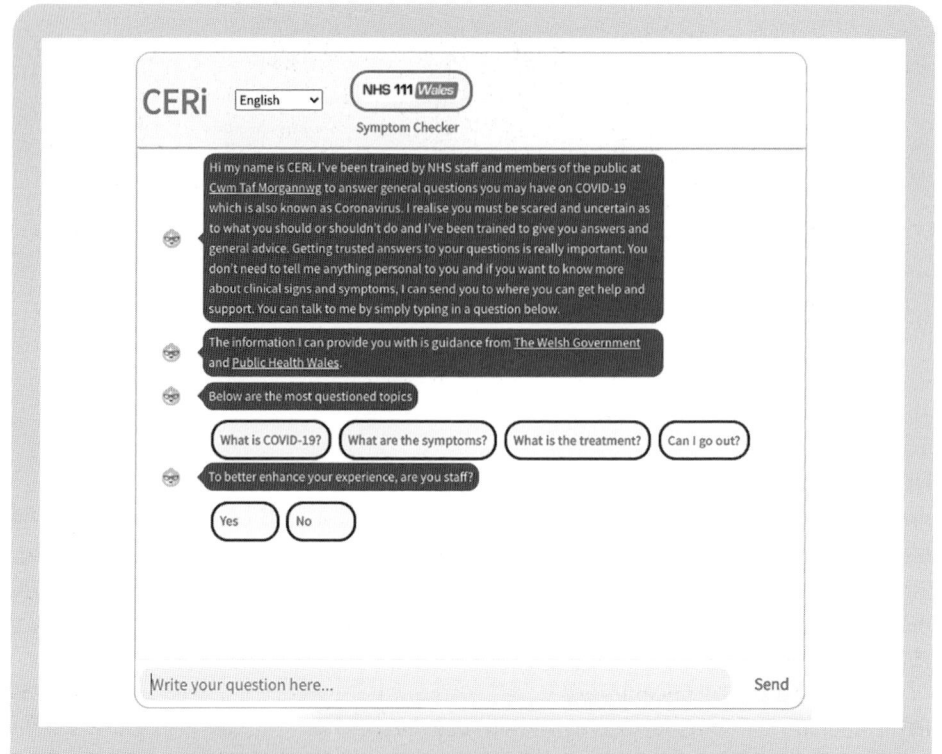

Figure 10.9: A preview of CERi, the IBM & NHS 111 artificial intelligence chatbot designed to reduce the personnel demand on NHS 111 staff during the COVID-19 pandemic.

Wearable Healthcare Technologies – 'Healthcare on the Go'
Smart Watches

Wearable technologies are becoming increasingly popular, with a 2019 survey recording 32.1% of the population now owning a smart watch. Step-counting, sleep tracking and heart rate monitoring can be carried out by smart watches and shared with the person's GP. However such information can also over-diagnose patients and be detrimental to their

> Using infra-red spectroscopy, smart watches can estimate a person's blood pressure through non-invasive means. Some technology also measures oxygen saturations. A third example of technological advancement is an electrocardiogram (ECG). For some patients, atrial fibrillation can last for a few minutes and be hard to identify clinically (as the heart may be in a normal sinus rhythm when attending a clinic). Smart watches with built in partial ECG technology can capture the episode and allow the patient to send this to their GP.

Figure 10.10: Smart Devices 1 - Observations.

> Fall detection is a significant concern, with approximately 30% of the 65+ population experiencing a fall each year. Falls cause fractures, risking the life, and ongoing quality of life. Some smart watches recognise falls using in-built 3D accelerometers, and some include an automated system whereby the wearer cannot dismiss the alert, and emergency services are automatically notified of the fall – with in-built GPS software to provide the location of the patient.

Figure 10.11: Smart Devices 2 - Falls.

well-being. The integration of data from smart devices into clinical decision-making requires significant further thought.

Wireless Continuous Observational Monitoring
Progress in wireless clinical observation is also taking place in secondary care. But it is important to note data from the two settings (primary and secondary) may require different interpretation. For example, in the community, a heart rate of 100 beats a minute may indicate a person is carrying out moderate exercise or carrying heavy shopping. However in a hospital, it may be indicative of a cardiovascular response to sepsis.

On hospital wards, nursing staff usually monitor patients every 4 hours, and feed this into National Early Warning Score (NEWS) paperwork. This is a non-specific measure of how unwell a patient is, and is used to detect patient deterioration. The nurses increase or decrease frequency of observations depending on the patient's clinical condition.

A recent UK trial explored the value of wireless, continuous monitoring of clinical observations during a hospital stay, to identify patient deterioration. Sensium, a company who specialise in wireless observational monitoring, created an adhesive waterproof patch which is placed on a patient's chest. The patch records their observations and notifies the clinical team of any changes.

3D Printed Prosthetics and Biomimetic Designs
Prosthetics have existed throughout human history. Indeed, a prosthetic eye was found in Iran in 3000-2800 BC. The development of prosthetics has evolved from wooden and metal products, through to refined plastics. Recently, with the use of Open-Source technology and 3D printers, prosthetic designers can upload their bespoke designs onto Open-Source libraries; allowing for people across the world to print them in any material compatible with 3D printers.

Prostheses themselves are also becoming more advanced. Dr Hugh Herr's team in MIT's Biomechatronics Research Group has created the world's first bionic lower limb - the BiOM Ankle. Their work aims to overcome issues with incumbent technology, such as failure to absorb the shock created by activity. This results in fatigue, limited activity and increased musculoskeletal problems.

Neuronal control of prosthetic limbs is also being developed by this team. Sensory nerves can be reconnected to regions near the amputation site; and with stimulation from pressure transducers on the prosthesis, sensory innervation can be interpreted. In other words, with the developments in both sensory and motor components of prostheses, it may be possible to develop artificial limbs that not only move because of thought, but also 'feel' the environment they are in.

Telemedicine – Healthcare in your Pocket
As a response to the C19 pandemic, GPs throughout the UK became reliant on telephone and video-based consultations. This form of consultation, whilst novel to the majority of NHS GPs, was already being used to increase access to primary healthcare.

For example, a primary healthcare company called Babylon started in London in 2013, providing largely virtual care for its patients. It was designed for younger, fitter patients, especially those who lived in large conurbations, i.e. those with episodic use, and reasonable digital access and competency. The service uses mobile devices to deliver video consultations with GPs, and will send prescriptions to local pharmacies for convenience. To access the service, patients only need to register through the mobile application, which is free to download.

Babylon operates well for uncomplicated, discrete health concerns. But it advises those who are frail, pregnant, have mental health concerns or complex healthcare needs, to stay with their current conventional general practice. Patients registering at Babylon currently have to de-register from their current GP, allowing for the transfer of their patient records. However, with closer IT interoperability in the future, services like Babylon may work with traditional GP services.

Smart Knives for Cancer Resection
Surgical resection requires clean margins around the tumour, to prevent cancerous tissue remaining in the body and continuing to proliferate. One technology being developed to aid this is the 'Smart Knife'.

The surgeon's blade heats up the tissue to create the incision, which creates an aerosol of molecules from the tissue being cut. The blade's in-built mass spectrometer gives instantaneous information to the surgeon, to identify whether the tissue is healthy or cancerous; reducing the chances of cancerous tissue being left in the body.

Surgical Training using Augmented Reality Technology
'Augmented reality' (AR) originates from the gaming industry and provides a mixed reality experience for the user. This mixed reality consists of the actual environment (the user is in) being incorporated into a 3D structure in the cyber-environment; visible through technology such as a phone screen or technology-enhanced eyewear. This technology has been assessed in a plethora of surgical specialities, including colorectal, orthopaedic, trauma and vascular surgery.

AR can provide surgical training, pre-operative surgical planning and intra-operative navigation. AR for surgical training may be preferred to the use of cadavers because of its ability to replicate the procedure; access technology in various educational settings, and in-built 'haptic feedback', which makes the experience more realistic.

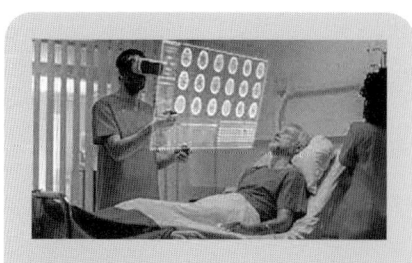

Figure 10.12: Augmented Reality on a Ward Round.

Virtual Patients

Virtual (computerised simulated) patients can be used for numerous aspects of clinical training: history-taking, communication skills, clinical science knowledge, professionalism - and even physical examination skills. Their use removes several barriers to clinical learning, such as a high volume of learners and not enough patients, or a lack of exposure to rarer diseases.

One study from the University of Warwick investigated the use of a 'longitudinal virtual patient' to train medical students' clinical reasoning - both in general practice and acute settings. Initial pilot data from the students was remarkably positive and the team is now exploring the possibility of creating several 'virtual patients'[22].

Benefits of Advances

The above examples are a glimpse into the future of technology that may have a significant impact on healthcare and health. However, the population that will benefit is still a relatively small one, compared to the wider NHS population. Also the method for spreading new technology is still limited. Thus the development of innovative, bespoke or niche technologies in one Trust may take considerable time to be rolled out.

Summary

The NHS is a world leading organisation in many ways. Its use of novel technology is no exception. But the NHS faces major challenges regarding raising the standard of its IT systems and devices.

In the future, patients will be empowered to engage with their own medical records and access services through their mobile devices. During the C19 pandemic, primary and secondary care adapted to increased and unprecedented demands in a short space of time, partly due to rapid IT advances. Nonetheless, there is a long way to go.

Further reading

Cancer Research UK: The intelligent knife: a potential 'game-changer' for cancer surgery.

https://news.cancerresearchuk.org/immersive-stories/the-intelligent-knife-a-potential-game-changer-for-cancer-surgery/

NHS: The Ambulance Response Programme home page.

https://www.england.nhs.uk/urgent-emergency-care/improving-ambulance-services/arp/

NHS Digital home page.

https://digital.nhs.uk/

NHS 'GP at Hand' home page.

https://www.england.nhs.uk/london/our-work/gp-at-hand-fact-sheet/

---

22. Yes, you may have your own cyber-patient to 'look after' for four or five years! They (and you) better get to clinic on time.

Chapter 11

Sorting out the NHS

"By the time you've sorted out a complicated idea into little steps that even a stupid machine can deal with, you've certainly learned something about it yourself". Douglas Adams, Dirk Gently's Holistic Detective Agency.

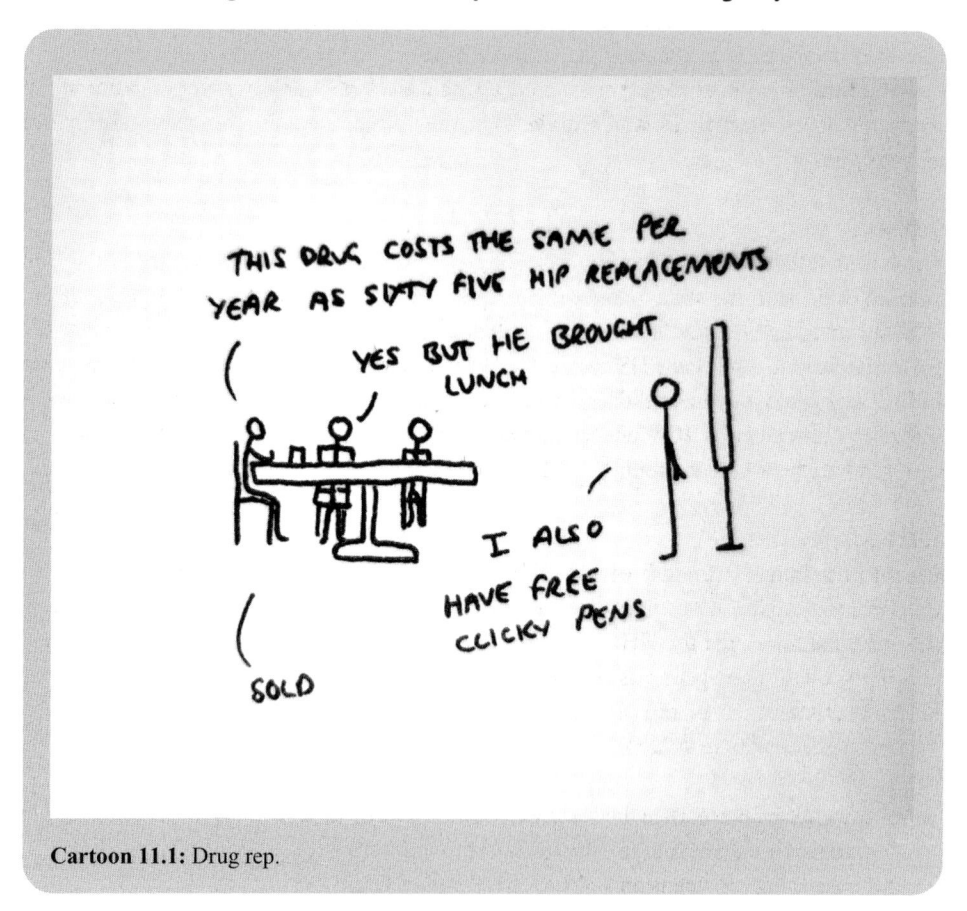

Cartoon 11.1: Drug rep.

Introduction
For the NHS to keep advancing, we need to be aware of its strengths and weaknesses. In the first section of this chapter, we start by identifying its five main strengths followed by its five biggest weaknesses, all of which need sorting. The second section attempts to answer (objectively) the question 'is the NHS any good?'

Five Biggest Strengths

National institution, and instrument of social change
The opening ceremony of the London 2012 Olympic Games included a homage to Britain's NHS. Creator Danny Boyle said:

> "it's something that we are really proud of. It celebrates something unique about this country".

He could have chosen some other aspect of society, like the BBC ('Auntie'), that we also feel affection for. Despite the failings of the NHS, even though the computers don't talk to each other, despite the parking, there is little doubt most of the British public share this affection, as we have seen during the C19 pandemic.

Its central role in our society may also be why it has been an instrument of major social change. A good example of which is the emancipation of women, through contraception and abortion, etc.

Politics
The NHS in 1948 was largely an NHS for England and Wales. Scotland and Northern Ireland were separate from the start. Wales separated fully later. These distinctions give each nation a feeling of pride in 'its NHS', as well as considerable control. NHS England (led by health professionals) took over the NHS in England in 2013 and acts as the principle 'provider' to the DHSC. In this way it is 'independent-ish' of government. This means we have been able to write a 5-year (2014) and now 10-year (2019) plan. There needs to be a long-term agreement (with cross party consensus) for a rolling 10-year plan, so it does not matter which party is in power.

Staff
Perhaps the biggest strength of the NHS is its staff. In most analyses of the worth of professions in the UK, doctors and nurses (and engineers and teachers) come out top. But we must not forget the NHS provides a very large number of reasonably or well-paid secure jobs with good pensions. A 'career' is not nothing. It is a great advantage in life to have a guaranteed salary and benefits, and a clear career ladder you can ascend.

One NHS employee said this recently, which sums it up:

> "I love to help people when they are most vulnerable. I cannot think of a more rewarding or worthwhile career. It is my way of contributing to the health and wellbeing of my local community which is one of the most deprived in the UK."

Funding
The NHS is a state funded service, where *funding is linked to population growth*. This is a simple statement but very important. It provides unusually good financial protection to the public from the consequences of ill health. In this way, it still provides the 1948 'Bevan-Attlee-Beveridge dream' of universal, equitable, comprehensive, good quality, free at the

point of delivery, and centrally-funded care[23]. And for all this, you pay nothing at the time, and no one bills you later.

It is also relatively cost-efficient. Being so large, it can buy in bulk. Hence the UK has the largest proportion of generic prescribing of all comparator countries: 84% in 2015, compared to an average of 50%. Also doctors are employed on salaries (hospital doctors) or by numbers of patients registered (GPs), rather than charging fees per procedure or per appointment. So there is no incentive to carry out unnecessary procedures or string out treatment. All of this is a huge advantage when compared to other systems.

Emphasis on primary care (especially general practice)
Why should I emphasise this part of the NHS staff? I am biased, as both my parents were GPs. I am writing these words in my Dad's chair from which he saw tens of thousands of patients over a long career. Nonetheless, and accepting that, I think GPs are special, and amongst the best bits of the NHS. I have no data to prove that. But I do have a lifetime of experience of primary, secondary, tertiary and other NHS care, and have been able to see all at close quarters.

The foundation of the NHS on a GP service, is in marked contrast with countries where the patient has direct access to specialists. The typical British GP in fact only refers about 5% of patients (per clinic) to hospitals every year. This means inappropriate and excessive use of hospital-based resources is minimised.

In general, private medicine encourages a concentration on specialisation to the neglect of general practice. This is certainly the case in France and Germany; and may be why Germany has three times our number of hospital beds per person, and Sweden less beds (see later). Also the UK (population 68 million) has the same number of ICU beds as Greece (10.4 million). This has caused concern during the C19 pandemic.

And it is also true that not all developed countries (e.g. USA) and emerging countries (e.g. India) have developed family doctor systems, and their health care is consequently poorer.

These five big strengths have not arisen by chance. Shoulders. Giants, etc. What will be your life mission? Add to, or consolidate, the five above? Or focus on a new one that you think should be on the list? Whatever you do, do it with passion and determination - and a bit of humour.

Five Biggest Areas for Improvement

These five areas have some common characteristics. They are important, connected, and in the 'too difficult box'. They are on all the risk registers. Each is left there festering, frustrating, and passed over (with a sigh) at repeating cycles of governance meetings.

Different governments have half-a-go at sorting a couple, then give in. All need to be sorted out to achieve a performance appropriate to a developed country, and allow us to call the NHS 'world class'[24]. Five years of a normal government term is not enough. To really sort them all will require the will of several government terms and all the staff of the

---

23. Read that out to yourself again. Pretty cool, eh?
24. AS does not know what 'world class' means. It's probably managerial twaddle that should be put in 'NHS Room 101' along with 'mission statements'.

NHS. The first four are, in our view, essential. Without sorting them, it will not advance. And they are not about money. On its own, money will not solve the NHS's problems.

Social

Warning. This bit is upsetting. It shows how we all have failed our elderly.

Social care is the biggest problem in care, and many would say in Western Culture, i.e. the lack of well-funded, joined up and compassionate health and social care. This is largely (but not exclusively) an issue for the frail elderly. The origin of this problem is found in the tripartite system of 1948, whereby social care was the responsibility of the council, and separate from the other two pillars of healthcare. It still is. Thus it remains grossly under-prioritised and under-funded. This encompasses care workers in the home, residential/nursing homes and day centres. It hugely affects the final years of life, perhaps yours. If it had affected the early years of life, maybe it would have been sorted.

If you are young(er) and think this is nothing to do with you, and not your fault, ask yourself this question. If your parent or grandparent became infirm and needed long term care 24/7, would you put your career on hold, move house, and move your children to a new school?

We often treat our frail elderly like irritating expensive cattle that need to be rehoused. Many other cultures, however, look after their frail elderly properly - with care, respect, dignity and love. We do not. We should hold our heads in shame.

The funding of most health and social care continues to be largely based in different government ministries, with different funding streams, computer systems, ambitions and priorities. Most healthcare comes from the Department of Health and Social Care (DHSC), but most adult social care comes from the local authority (i.e. originally from the Department for Levelling Up, Housing and Communities (DLUHC)). It is a misnomer to

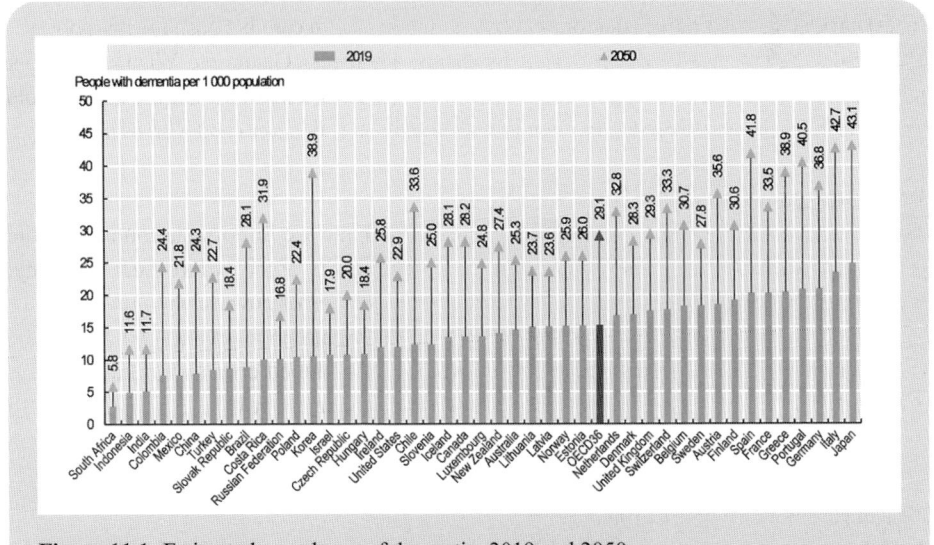

Figure 11.1: Estimated prevalence of dementia, 2019 and 2050.

say that the Department of Health and *Social Care* is fully responsible for social, when it does not fund most of it, and does not run it.

It is essential, as a caring society, to keep disadvantaged, frail and elderly people well and living independently - and out of hospital. This issue was obvious during the first wave of C19 when the NHS knowingly sent infectious (untested) patients back to residential homes, causing multiple outbreaks and death. We are all to blame for this mistake.

These issues will get worse, for two reasons. Firstly, we know the dementia epidemic is already here, and will get worse (see Figure 11.1). Secondly, the proportion of older people in society is increasing markedly (see Figure 11.2). Neither issue will go away. Their relative share of funding is shown in Figure 11.3.

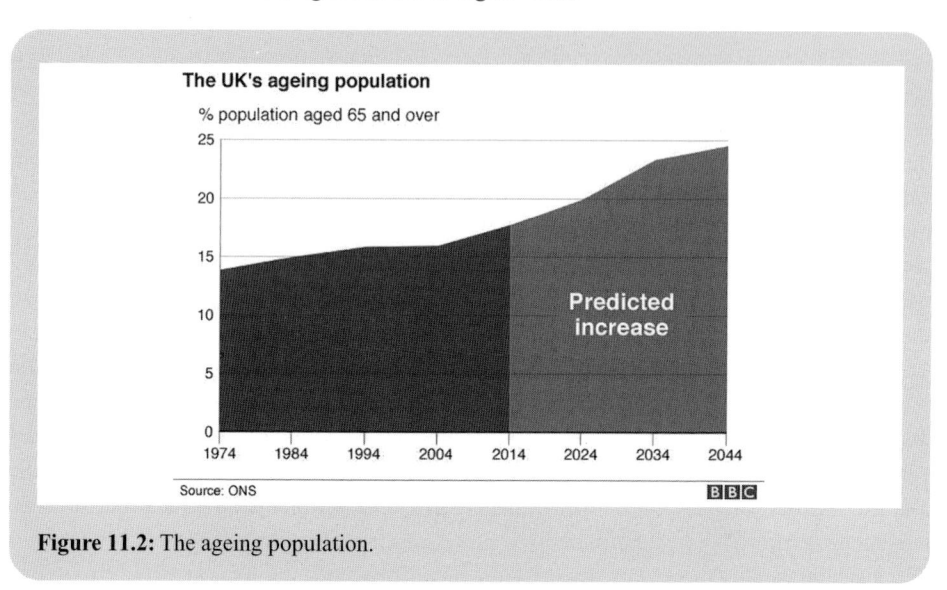

Figure 11.2: The ageing population.

Figure 11.3: Relative funding of health and social care.

What is the answer? We need a cross-party consensus, and the public will need to pay more through general taxation to support social care. If we do not, hospitals will continue to be jammed, targets missed, waiting lists lengthen, and there will be continued misery for the frail and elderly. It is our moral duty to sort it out.

This is why personalised budgets (mentioned in Chapter 12) may help. It costs less to provide care for elderly patients in their own home, than paying for care homes and having elderly people in acute hospitals unnecessarily. These are the approximate comparative costs of long-term healthcare:

1. Home   £60-120/day (4 x 30-60 mins. visits by support worker)
2. Nursing/residential home   £150 a day
3. Hospital   £400 a day.

Seven Day NHS and Social Care
Patients get ill and need healthcare every day of the week. Why would there be less cases of appendicitis at the weekend? The NHS and the administration of social care work 5 days a week. Previous efforts to make them seven-day service (7DS) have largely failed. We need to try again.

If we do not, then chaos will continue with emergency patients continuing to pour into hospitals over the weekend, whilst we discharge relatively few (about 60% of normal on a Saturday, 40% on Sunday). We cannot discharge patients to residential/nursing homes at the weekend nor arrange care workers in the home. So, on Mondays, hospitals cancel elective surgery, as 'beds are full' (yes, again[25]), and GPs come into excessive workloads. It is a Kafka-esque repeating nightmare.

Furthermore, there is an 11% increase in mortality if you are admitted to hospital on a Saturday, Sunday or Bank Holiday – no matter if it is for emergency or elective care, or whether you are high, medium or low risk. Tesco, and other supermarkets, work seven-days a week. The NHS will have to be a 7DS one day. So we might as well do it now.

But do we have staff to provide a similar NHS seven days a week? Maybe, maybe not. Answer? Rotas (see below). If hospitals provide a 7DS, then GPs should do - as should community physios, pharmacists and social care. We are all in this together, otherwise it is pointless.

Within hospitals, a simple solution is to 'do a Tesco' and run the NHS with two four-day teams, Monday-Thursday, and Thursday-Sunday, with Thursday being the handover day - 10-hour days, four days a week, 40 hours, bosh. Teams swap around every 4 months (to coincide with the change of junior doctors). It is possible, if rotas are clever, and average staff numbers need not be much lower than in the current five-day week.

Elective vs emergency care – failure to separate
Two of the strengths of the NHS are that in an emergency you will be treated immediately, and if you have a long-term condition, you will be treated until it is cured, or controlled. But

---

25. Yes, it is Groundhog Day.
    Again...

if you need a hip replacement, you may have to live in pain, even if you are incapacitated, sometimes for months before you have effective treatment (which by then is less effective). Similarly, if you need a cataract operation, you may remain blind unnecessarily for months. In June 2021, 5.5 million people in England were on some form of NHS waiting list, one in 10 of the population.

Why is this? It is largely a product of the combination of a lack of 7DS and the failure to separate elective and emergency care. Why? We will always, naturally, favour a newly confused frail elderly lady with a UTI and/or social problems, over a planned operation on Monday. The operation - which may be a cancer or vital heart operation - gets postponed (again). This is understandable but is it right?

Answer. We need to fully separate elective and emergency care and place them in different locations - and run them as 7DS. Easier said than done.

Integration, Geography and Information Technology
Healthcare, social care, geography and IT are connected. Or rather they are not. That's the problem. Problems 1-3 above fall out of this lack of integration. True integration cannot occur until we have coterminous entities with common IT systems, and a single Government department 'in charge' and a national (population based) funding system

Back to IT. Why is it so important? Because it is a big part of the solution. The NHS (and social care) have a fundamental lack of a common coterminous IT system, and thus the means to share information. The last attempt at a national electronic patient record (EPR) has been abandoned. Primary care, secondary care, mental health, and the ambulance service (and other parts of the NHS) use different (often incompatible) IT systems, working across (i.e. not with) different regional geographical patches. Social care and public health are entities on another IT planet.

They act in silos which are unaware of what the other silos are doing. This is so frustrating when you know that thing or person you need to 'talk to' is 'out there' (and may be down the corridor) but you are unable to contact it or them. And vice versa. But sub-regional EPRs are starting to happen (probably based on the 42 ICSs). They will be expensive but so be it. This needs to be a high priority, and NHS Digital/X needs to drive this, and make sure they are compatible, then link them up at a national level.

There are currently plans to further integrate primary, secondary and tertiary healthcare, with social care, via the ICS system. We think this is a 'good' thing, and the NHS is moving in the right direction. EPRs will be very important and will 'bind' ICSs together. But these will have limited effect unless we deal with:
1. Full financial (and organisational) integration. This will require an Act of Parliament, to 'move' social care from DLUHC (council) to the DHSC (NHS) and decide how it will be paid for. But, at the time of writing, with a white paper published concerning the ICS reforms, this does not appear to be a priority. As such, it is possible the (generally good) formation of ICSs (that are probably the 'right-size') will have little long-term benefit as they ignore the bigger issues, and are not geographically coterminous. This leads us on to…

2. Nitty-gritty problems. These are described above and currently in the 'too difficult box', i.e. 7DS and separating elective and emergency care.
3. Geography. Change it, it's possible.

Lack of Coterminous Structures
We have one NHSE, with its 7 regions and will have 42 ICSs (based on an unknown and changing number of CCGs). They will loosely 'work with' but are not part of 13 LETBs (part of HEE), 14 ambulance trusts, four public health regions (and 8 centres), 24 county and 333 local councils. It is mad. There are historical reasons for this chaos. 400+ years of stable democracy is good for democracy (as no one has too much power) but does not help the organisation and integration of healthcare, public health and social care.

Answer (to all of this) – Our 7 Point Plan
If one was designing a country, one would not have come up with the above systems in what we now call 'England' or the 'UK', or the National *Health* Service.

So what is the solution? What would it look like, this 'perfect health/social care in England/UK'?
1. Healthcare. One subregional (ICS-size) and regional entity (to include it all, e.g. ambulances, Research, Health & Justice 'services' etc.)
2. Social care. Same subregional and regional entity
3. Public Health. Same subregional and regional entity
4. IT, joining up 1, 2 and 3. Same subregional and regional entity (with national compatibility)
5. NHS 'takes over' (or at least, truly works with) social care. Run a 7DS
6. Separate elective and emergency care. Run a 7DS in both – i.e. routine operations and clinics as normal at weekends, as well as emergencies
7. All within the same population-based funding body (reporting to one government ministry, ideally DHSC); that has to keep within budget by law, like councils. That they do not just leads to loose accounting, and a lack of public debate regarding priority setting.

Not easy we know. But a lot of other issues would be simpler if we could rewrite history and geography!

Other Stuff – Data Protection, Quality and Choice
This section raises questions about data security and rights of access, but it must be better than the current situation of poor or non-existent communication - some of it on paper - which is costing lives.

It is not just communication within the NHS, it's information regarding the quality of care we all need. We can find more about the quality and origin of tomatoes in Sainsbury's, than patients can find about how good or bad a particular doctor is - let alone basic mortality figures. So there is little real freedom, and no real choice, in making healthcare decisions. This is a situation that only good IT systems can overturn.

Performance
This point is a consequence of the four issues already discussed.

The performance of the NHS is judged by its key performance indicators (KPIs). Solve the four issues above, and it would fly. Below is the current state of play regarding some of those KPIs. It does not make easy reading. It is the fault of us all, not the government, 'the Trust', the authorities. It is the responsibility of all of us to sort it out. If we do not, the NHS will be jammed, inefficient, frustrating and chaotic forever. How are we doing? Not great.

In July 2021, 77.7% of people attending A&E spent less than four hours from arrival to admission, transfer or discharge. The target is over 95% - not achieved since July 2015.

As at the end of October 2021, 65.6% of patients had their first treatment in secondary care in 18 weeks (Referral to Treatment, RTT) or less. The current target is 92% - not achieved since in February 2016.

In June 2021, 73.3% of patients started their first treatment for cancer following an urgent GP referral in less than two months (62-day target). The current target is 85% - not achieved since December 2015. C19 has significantly worsened RTT and cancer treatment performance.

It is not clear why there are no easily accessible key performance indicators for general practice, dentistry or optometry. There should be.

International Comparisons – How good is the NHS?
Saying things like 'the NHS is the best health service in the world' or the 'NHS is world class' is not helpful. Stating any country has that title without supporting data is untrue.

What is true? Do these performance issues matter? Is the NHS any good? Do our KPIs matter? If not, what should be used to judge performance? Is our country any different from other developed countries in terms of healthcare? These are hard questions to answer[26].

Probably the best way of answering that question is Organisation for Economic Co-operation and Development (OECD) data. The OECD is an intergovernmental economic organisation with 37 members. It intermittently produces 'Health at a Glance', the last time being 2019, which compares key indicators for population health and health system performance across OECD countries.

It highlights how countries differ in terms of the health status and health-seeking behaviour of their citizens. It looks at access to, and quality of, health care and the resources available. It is probably the best way to look at the NHS objectively, and compare it to other similar countries, and answer the fundamental questions like 'is it any good' or 'is it well staffed and funded?'

---

26. There are deeper ones too. For example, is 'health' more important than 'education'? Which should be receiving more funding, etc.? Most health inequality is due to lack of education.

Overall
Infant Mortality

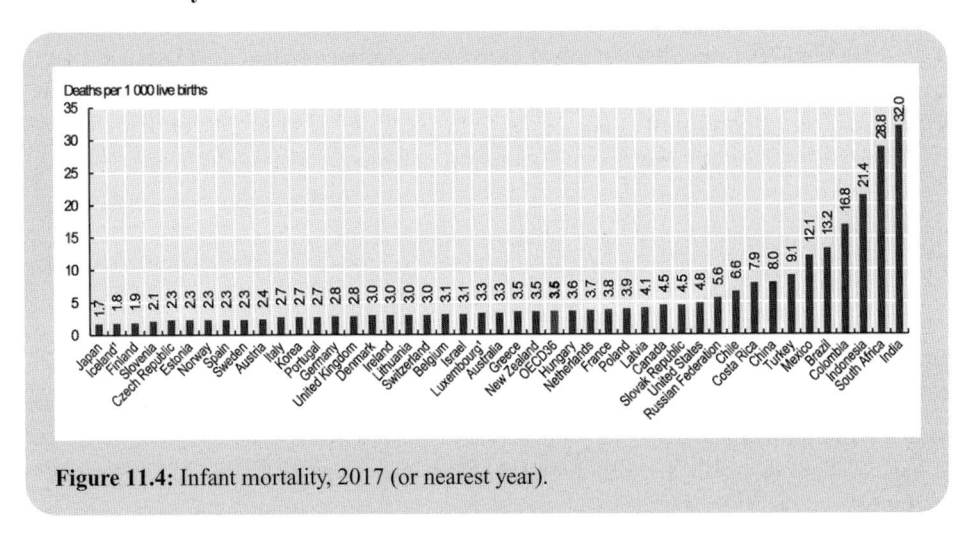

Figure 11.4: Infant mortality, 2017 (or nearest year).

Conclusion. Infant mortality is considered one of the best markers of the overall efficacy of healthcare systems - the UK is better than average.

Cancer Mortality

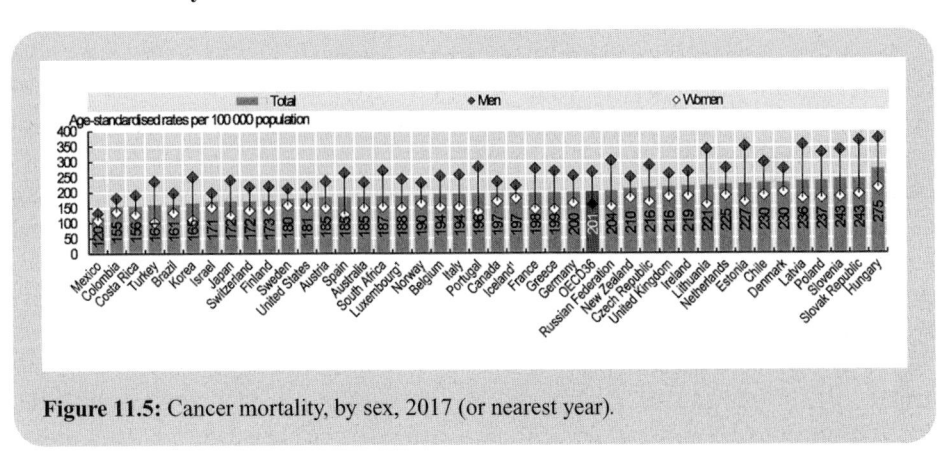

Figure 11.5: Cancer mortality, by sex, 2017 (or nearest year).

Conclusion. Cancer mortality is another marker of the overall efficacy of healthcare systems. There is no international data to compare the 62-day cancer performance indicator. But the mortality from cancer may be a reasonable surrogate for that – the UK performs OK.

On the other hand, if the UK is seen as one of the European countries, we have one of the worst cancer mortality figures. This is perhaps because we lack 170 oncologists, with a predicted shortage of about 230 oncologists by 2023. We also lack cancer nurses and therapeutic radiographers, and access to radiotherapy treatment is variable (poor in more remote settings).

Life Expectancy

Figure 11.6: Life expectancy at age 65, 1970 and 2017 (or nearest year).

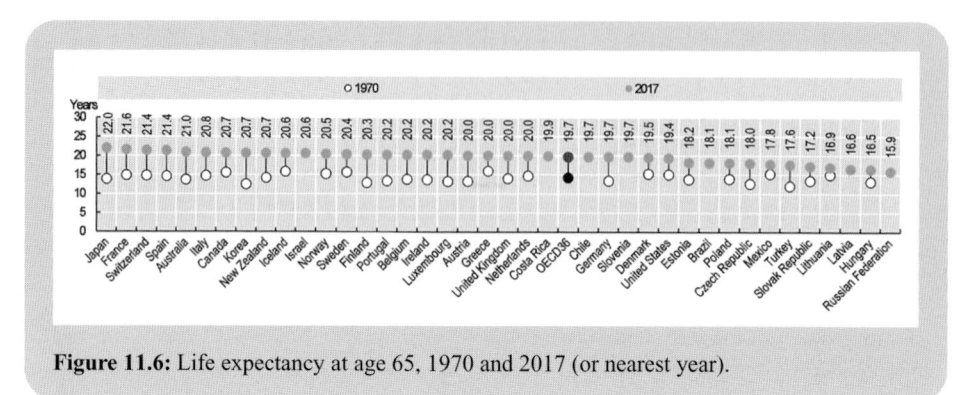

Conclusion. Most healthcare is delivered in the last 10-15 years of life. In terms of life expectancy, the UK is average and improving. If you get to 65 years, you are likely to live another twenty years on average.

Primary Care
Contacts with Doctors

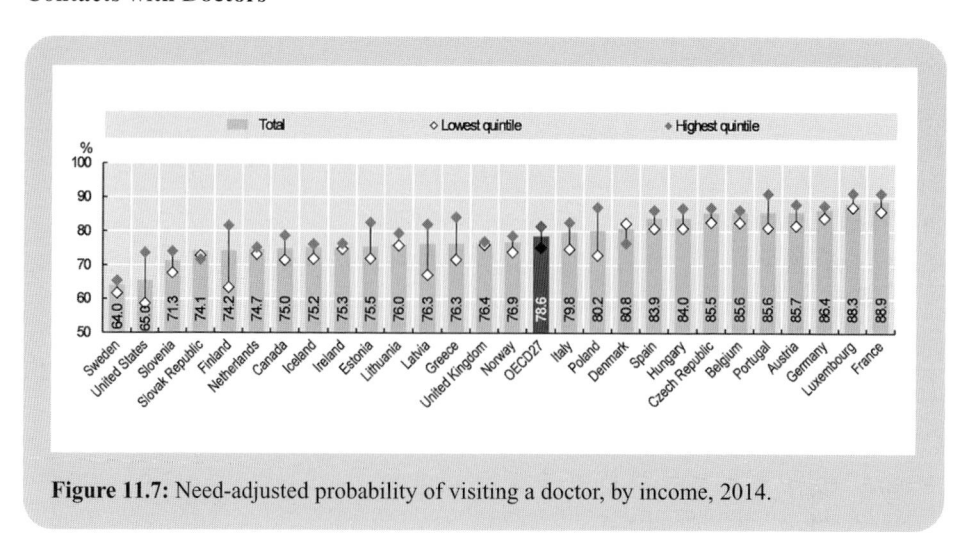

Figure 11.7: Need-adjusted probability of visiting a doctor, by income, 2014.

Conclusion. This data is for all contacts with doctors. But as most first contacts are with GPs, this table largely relates to them - UK citizens seem no more or less likely to visit a doctor than average.

Vaccination

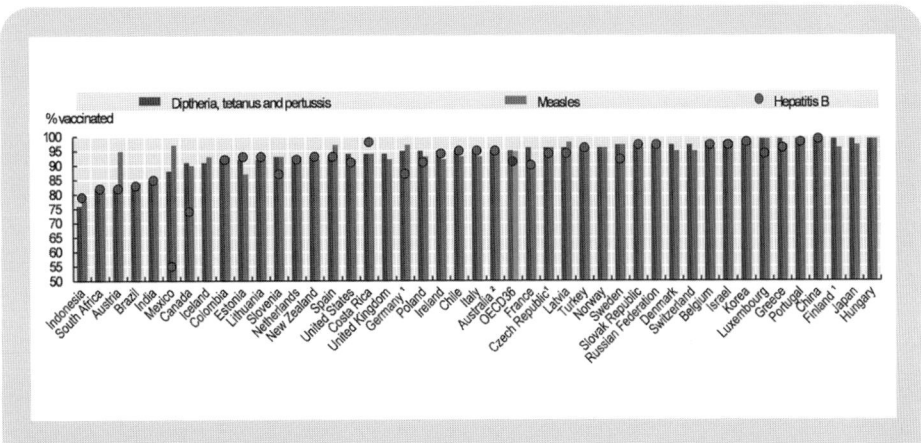

Figure 11.8: Percentage of children at 1 year of age vaccinated for diphtheria, tetanus and pertussis (DTP), measles and hepatitis B, 2018 (or nearest year).

Conclusion. A combination of public health and GP services leads to an average performance regarding vaccination. So far, it is (well, was) better than average re C19.

Secondary Care
Myocardial Infarction Mortality

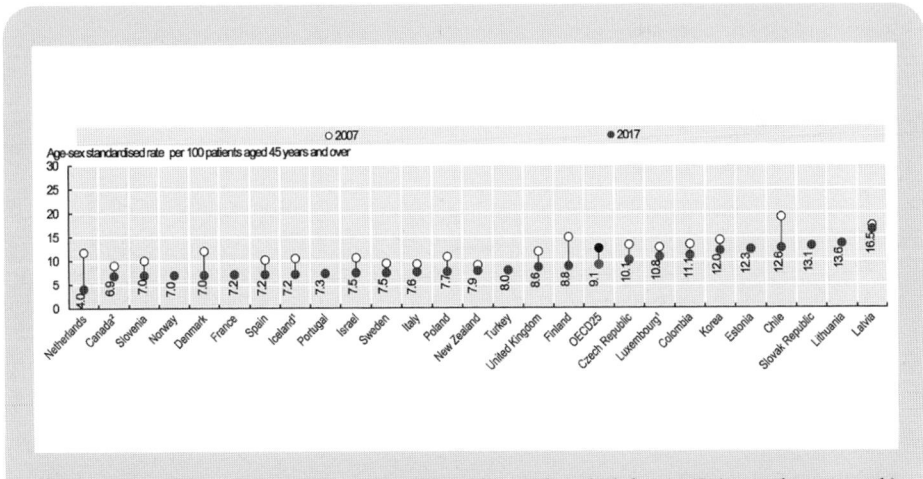

Figure 11.9: Thirty-day mortality after admission to hospital for AMI (acute heart attack) based on linked data, 2007 and 2017 (or nearest year).

Conclusion. Mortality from acute myocardial infarction (AMI) may be a reasonable surrogate for the A&E four hour wait target – the UK is average and improving.

Hip Replacements

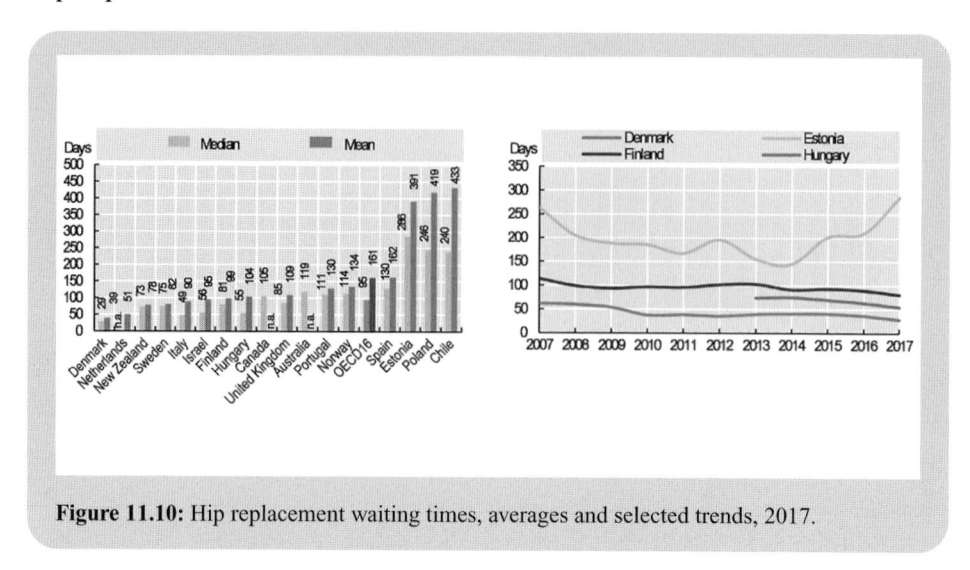

Figure 11.10: Hip replacement waiting times, averages and selected trends, 2017.

Conclusion. Hip replacement waiting times may be a reasonable surrogate for the 18-week RTT – the UK, again, is OK.

Mental Health
Suicide

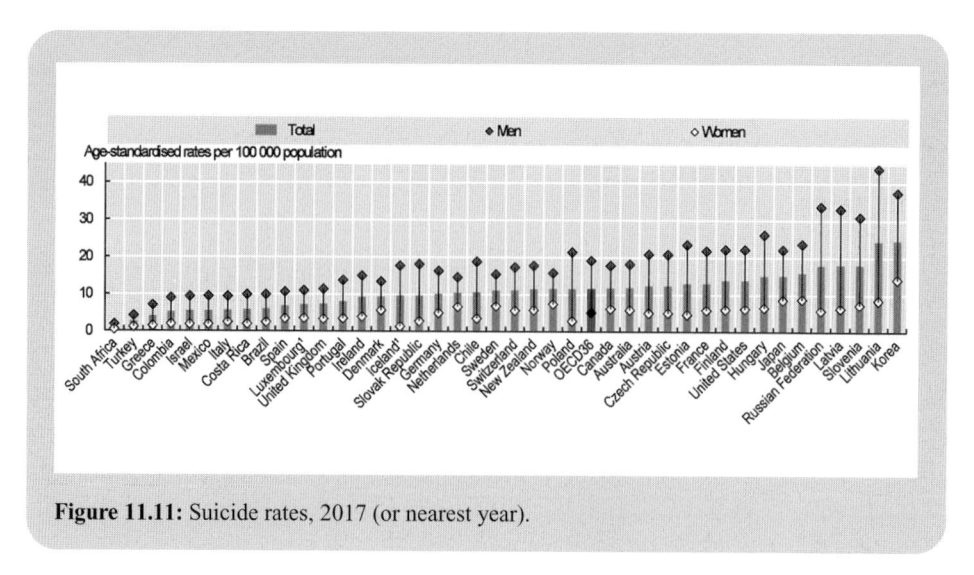

Figure 11.11: Suicide rates, 2017 (or nearest year).

Conclusion. Suicide is a surrogate for our mental health targets – the UK is doing better than average.

Staffing
Number of Doctors

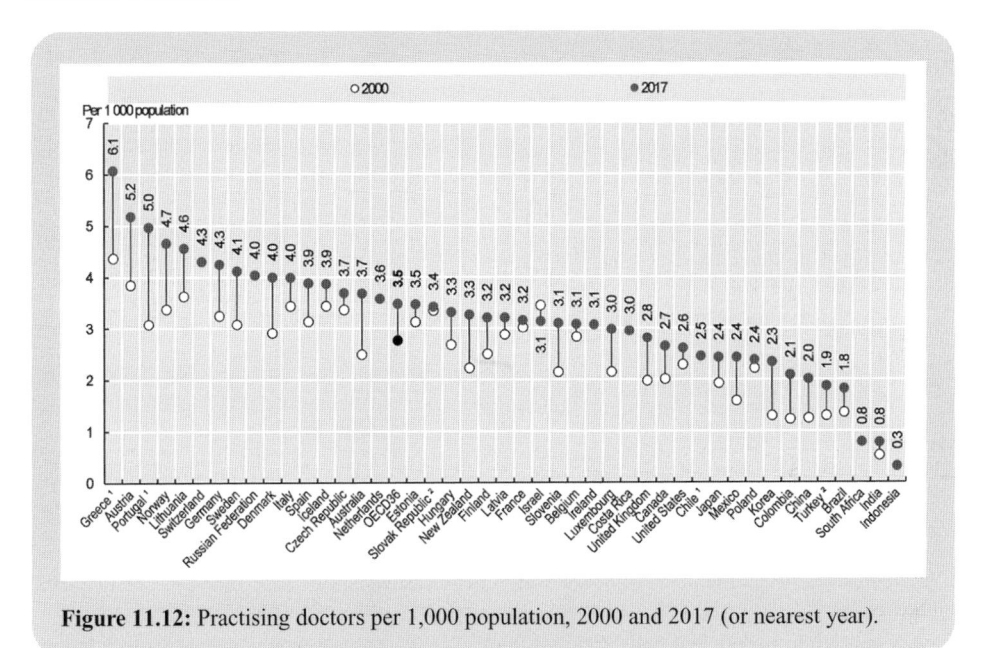

Figure 11.12: Practising doctors per 1,000 population, 2000 and 2017 (or nearest year).

Conclusion. This data provides some evidence to support the view there are 'not enough doctors' in the UK. The numbers are, however, rising.

Number of Nurses

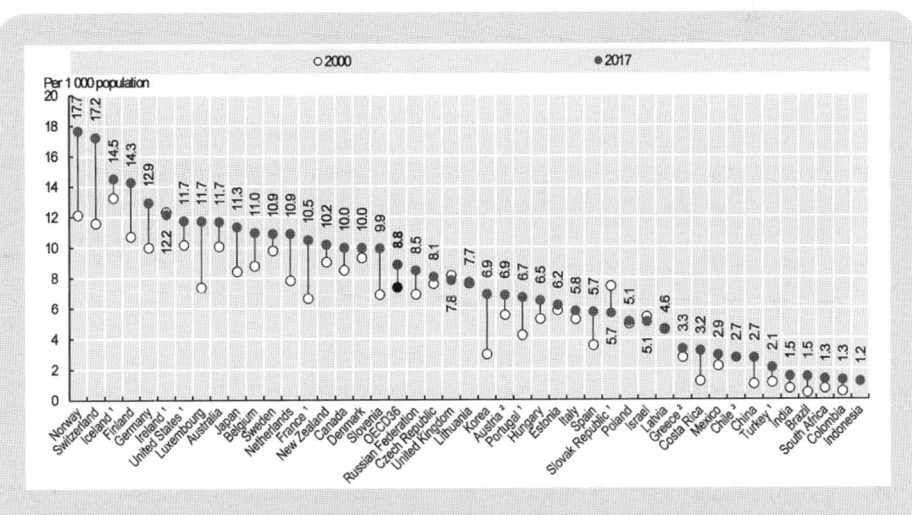

Figure 11.13: Practising nurses per 1,000 population, 2000 and 2017 (or nearest year).

Conclusion. There is also a widespread belief that there are 'not enough nurses' – in fact, the UK has an average number.

Facilities, Efficiency and Costs
Bed Numbers

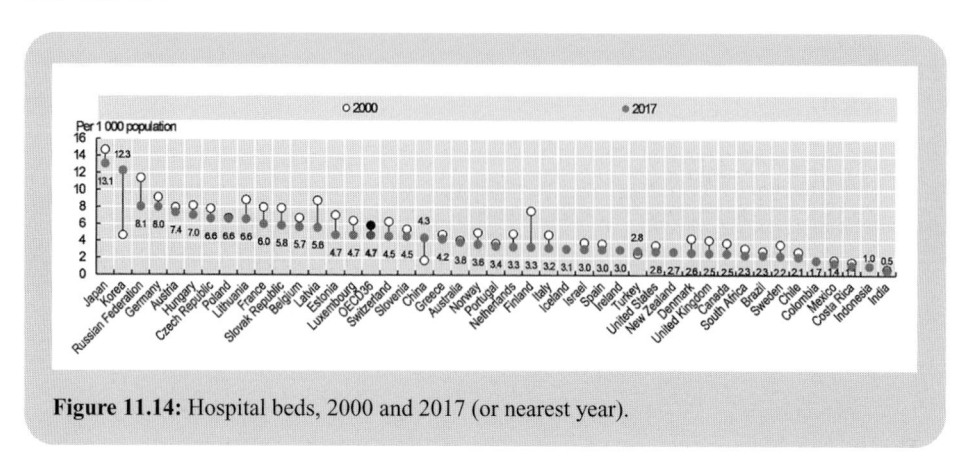

Figure 11.14: Hospital beds, 2000 and 2017 (or nearest year).

Conclusion. There is also a widespread view that the NHS does 'not have enough beds' – the UK has a low number of beds and less than in 2000. However we do have a more active primary care system than most countries.

Hospital Length of Stay

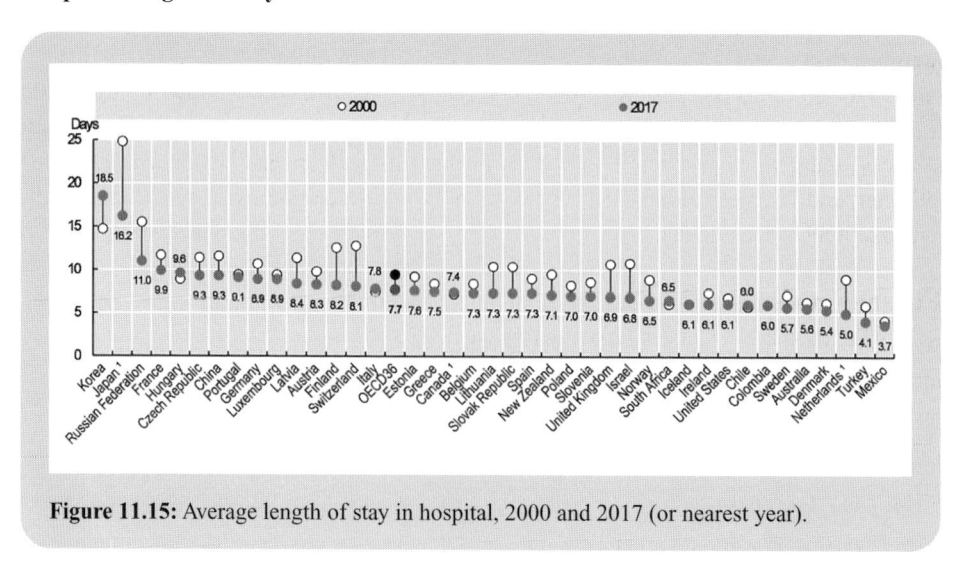

Figure 11.15: Average length of stay in hospital, 2000 and 2017 (or nearest year).

Conclusion. We seem to use those beds wisely and efficiently, with an average length of stay of 6.9 days and falling.

Spending

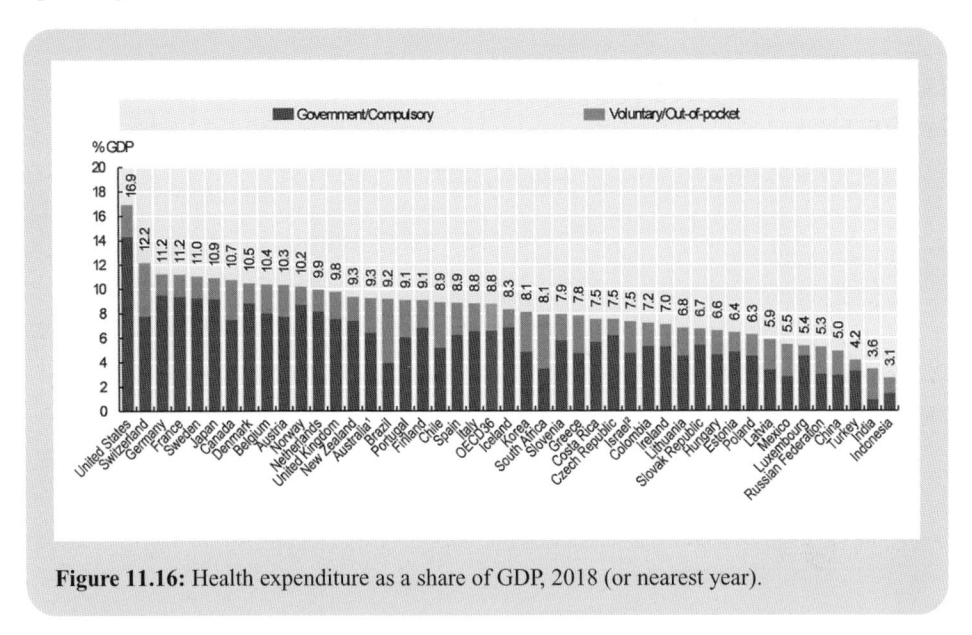

Figure 11.16: Health expenditure as a share of GDP, 2018 (or nearest year).

Conclusion. Our national spending on the NHS is better (9.8% of GDP) than the international average. Most people feel that the NHS needs more money. So long as the link to population growth continues, it may not need a huge amount more.

Overall Conclusion

So, what is the final conclusion? After 70 years+ of development is it any good? It is the view of the author that the NHS is quite good, and good value for money. Let's say, overall, it is a 'C+' ('B-' on a good day). 'A' for some things. It is better at acute and maternity services, and general practice; less good at planned surgery, mental health (especially for children) and IT/integration (especially with social care). It is your role to 'finish the job' and take it all to excellence.

Further reading

King's Fund: The NHS at 70: How good is the NHS?

https://www.kingsfund.org.uk/publications/nhs-70-how-good-is-the-nhs

NHS: Five-year forward view.

https://www.england.nhs.uk/five-year-forward-view/

NHS: Long term plan.

https://www.longtermplan.nhs.uk/

NHS: Statistics work areas.

https://www.england.nhs.uk/statistics/statistical-work-areas/

Nuffield Trust: NHS receives mixed scorecard in major analysis of international health systems.
https://www.nuffieldtrust.org.uk/news-item/nhs-receives-mixed-scorecard-in-major-analysis-of-international-health-systems

Organisation for Economic Co-operation and Development: Health at a Glance 2019.
https://www.oecd.org/health/health-systems/health-at-a-glance-19991312.htm

Chapter 12

The Future of the NHS

"The past is written, but the future is left for us to write." Jean-Luc Picard

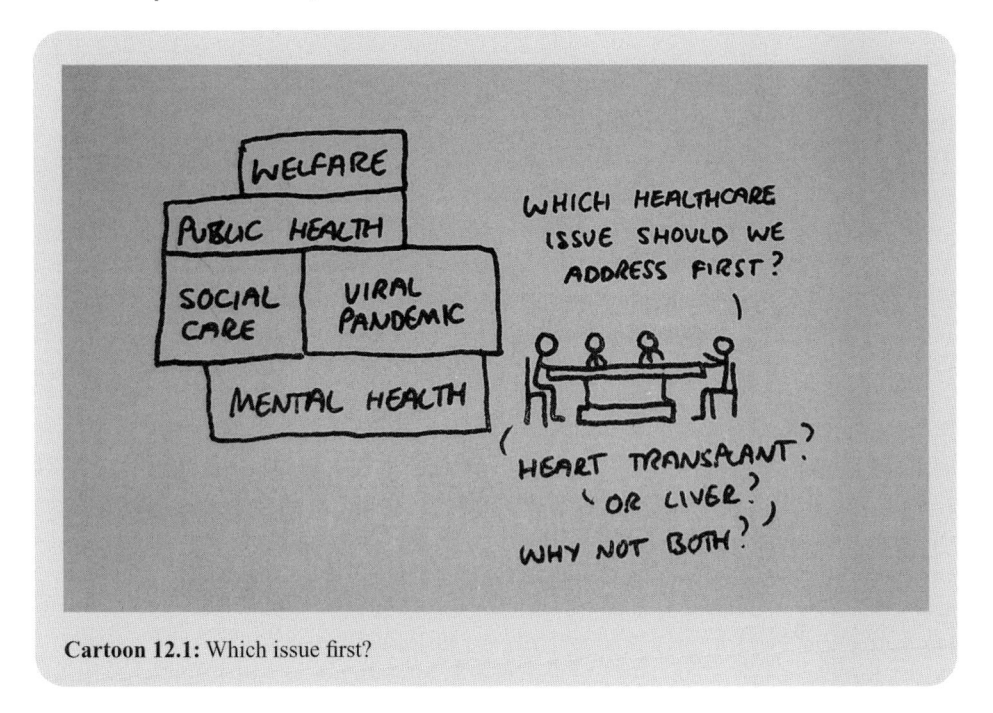

Cartoon 12.1: Which issue first?

Predictions

The only certainty we have is any prediction of the future will be wrong. For example, 'young people' would find it difficult to believe there was a time before the T-shirt. In the 1950s, it was merely an American version of the vest. Was there life before the rucksack? How many of us could have imagined the Berlin Wall coming down in 1989? Or the C19 pandemic?

This chapter attempts to predict the unpredictable. Only time will tell whether we have got any of it right. It is important in such discussions to set the bar high – e.g. is the NHS good enough for your Mum, now or in the future?

Background

The NHS Constitution (first published in 2009) restated its original values, which have survived through key reforms in the late '80s and early 2000s: offering comprehensive and excellent care to all, according to need and not based on ability to pay.

The NHS has been resilient, changing regularly, often to the frustration of staff. In recent years, it has also formed strong partnerships with private providers resulting in thousands of elective operations happening each year in private hospitals via 'choose and book'. This is understandably controversial, especially as just over 7% of the healthcare budget goes to private providers, up 2% since 2011-12.

This model of care has offered patients more choice for treatment location, increased competition amongst hospitals and reduced the burden of planned non-urgent surgery on the NHS (which can invest in more urgent care). Other private organisations have also won contracts to run essential NHS community services and urgent care centres across the UK - in a true 'public-private' collaborative model of care. This is not always popular as it seems to be in contradiction to its founding principles.

Surgical and Multidisciplinary Practice

The Calman-Hine report in 2015 uncovered unacceptable surgical practice variation in cancer care across the UK, resulting in poorer cancer patient outcomes. This led to the development of managed clinical networks, whereby professionals of different types (e.g. surgeons, physicians, pathologists and radiologists: often from different hospitals) provide joint consultations and shared learning. Multidisciplinary team meetings became clinical forums for reaching consensus, e.g. cancer or dialysis/renal transplantation - and remain the cornerstone of complex disease practice.

NHS Plans

The NHS intermittently produces long-term plans. The NHS Five Year Forward View (5YFV) in 2014, advocated greater investment in cancer, mental health, and primary care services. It supported greater inter-organisational collaboration between these, and community services - whilst advocating increased patient control. In 2015, 50 'vanguard' areas began to develop and evaluate the proposed care model. At the same time, the government invested in programmes such as 'Realising the Value' and the 'NHS Test Beds'; bringing in the voluntary and commercial/technology sectors. Social prescribing, which relied on collaboration between primary care and the voluntary sector, attempted to reduce the pressures on primary and specialist care.

The NHS Long Term Plan (LTP), published in January 2019, proposed a more personalised healthcare approach. This offered more choice and ensured the right treatment is given at the right time - hopefully leading to improved clinical outcomes. 42 sub-regional Integrated Care Systems (ICS) have been established across England, each covering a population of over 1 million people. They comprise mergers of 'purchasers' (e.g. CCGs) and 'providers' (e.g. GPs and hospitals). It will require an Act of Parliament to give them statutory status, combine budgets and have clear responsibility for care. This is happening at present.

Their formation will start to dismantle the 'internal market' of the early 1980s. They should transfer investment to primary, community, and voluntary services; hopefully with priorities set by multi-professional local Primary Care Networks (PCNs, i.e. groups of GP practices). Ideally, they will be formally incorporated into the ICSs. GP involvement is vital because they are 'nearer to the people' (hopefully 'speaking for the people'), and so recognise their current and future needs.

Ageing Population

The NHS is undoubtedly facing significant challenges due to the ageing population, and the higher cost of chronic illness. But, as stated previously, the UK spending on healthcare is similar to other developed countries as a percentage of GDP. The cost of chronic illness and ageing is derived from expensive treatments, increasing hospital admissions with longer lengths of stay, longer waits in EDs and increasing mental healthcare costs.

Population health challenges such as cardiovascular disease, stroke and cancer are still the major causes of mortality in the UK. All have reversible risk factors such as obesity, smoking, poor diet, and lack of exercise. Integrated Care Systems (ICSs) are uniquely placed to address such lifestyle choices.

Digital Opportunities

Matt Hancock MP, the former Minister of Health and Social Care, stated the NHS is best placed to become the most technically advanced healthcare system in the world, e.g. supported by digital and technological transformation. The creation of sub-regional EPRs should lead to a near complete clinical record, linking primary, secondary, and other (e.g. mental health) care information. In most areas of the UK, these records are not currently linked leading to clinical errors, and frustration for both patients and health professionals. Also, population data and data analytics (from EPRs) can drive research and development, leading to new treatments and new models of care.

Defining the New Vision for the NHS

The NHS prides itself for being one of the first healthcare systems in the world which is free at the point of need. The NHS Constitution mission statement includes this fundamental premise:

> "The NHS belongs to the people and communities it serves; its duty is to provide high quality and comprehensive care at best value and be accountable to people. Access to NHS services is based on clinical need, not an individual's ability to pay".

These high ambitions are as true now as they were in 1948. In the grand scheme however, it is not cheap and nor is it free (it needs 9% of your hard-earned taxes).

The future financial sustainability of the NHS depends on the adoption of a clear vision by all stakeholders, including patients and healthcare professionals. It may not be enough to aim for the NHS to be just the safest; it needs to be the most innovative healthcare system in the world. The ability to offer high quality, equitable and effective services to people will require considerable investment in estates, workforce numbers, partnerships, innovation and technology.

Innovation

The search for novel models of care and services is not necessarily synonymous with high cost. Indeed innovation can reduce healthcare costs. By engaging in innovation, the

NHS will continue to attract an innovative workforce, who can innovate to achieve cost efficiencies and better models of care.

Data
The collection and analysis of Real-World Data (RWD) - such as patient-reported outcome measures (PROMs), patient-reported experience measures (PREMs) and long-term clinical outcomes (e.g. quality-of-life), should pave the way towards personalised care. In addition, the use of digital technologies, e.g. patient portals and apps, can maximise RWD collection from patients remotely. The systematic collection of RWD can inform us better about population health and clinical performance, leading to more appropriate allocation of healthcare resources and budgets.

Leadership
The key to achieving the above vision lies in strong medical and clinical leadership. Leadership should not just be top-down but should be in partnership with local and regional communities, who should take control of their health, possibly through ICSs and PCNs. The role of local and regional medical directors is fundamental to implementing the NHS vision, through continuous engagement with their professional colleagues and patients. Doctors and nurses are leaders and subject matter experts, so their presence in positions of influence should increase. They should be supported by training and mentorship from senior NHS leaders. The future NHS should be a clinically-led healthcare system.

NHS Corporate Social Responsibility
People
The Interim NHS People Plan was first published in June 2019 and advocates equality and diversity in the workforce, as well as equal opportunities for development and promotion in the future NHS. Improving clinical outcomes and patient experience is paramount and cannot be compromised, even if evolving technology and automation leads to less personal interactions. All health professionals must learn new skills such as more careful history taking on the phone (e.g. without non-verbal communication, but with patient mobile phone photography, video assessment) and deciding who to bring to the surgery, or hospital, for physical examination.

Achieving this will require strong clinical leadership and creation of an innovative multi-professional and multi-cultural workforce; giving increased responsibility to non-medical staff such as clinical nurse specialists, advanced practitioners, pharmacy prescribers, physician associates and IT leads. The high demand for complex and specialist care means the current workforce needs to grow, as well as diversify. More engagement between senior managers and frontline NHS staff will empower strategic and innovative thinking. This will optimise adoption and implementation of new models of care, e.g. more community care and leveraging digital technology.

Community education about lifestyle change, health promotion and social prescribing can empower people to self-manage their long-term conditions and seek appropriate help. For example, for patients who suffer from seasonal depression, social prescribing (talking therapy and group exercise) can make a big difference.

'Social Movement' and Education

In addition, communities who volunteer to help and motivate each other to make healthier food choices, take regular exercise, stop smoking and reduce alcohol intake, could reduce attendances to primary and secondary care[27]. The 5YFV (2015) and the LTP (2019) set out the vision for the NHS as a 'social movement', underlining that the financial sustainability of the NHS depends on communities taking greater control over their health.

But. Hold on there. Us lot ('health') can be over earnest in terms of our social importance (and thus need for money). A complex modern society needs education, local government, transport, defence, and law and order, not just health. So health professionals need to live within their budget and not constantly ask central government for more money.

Furthermore educating young people out of 'cycles of deprivation' is far more effective in terms of preventing disease, than patching adults up when disease is established.

Environment

The NHS has a responsibility towards the environment. A lot can be done in this area; from building NHS estates using sustainable materials, to refurbishing old buildings, and using technology to achieve energy efficiency. C19 has led to a rapid increase in virtual appointments dramatically reducing the need for travel - so reducing health's carbon footprint.

Brexit and the NHS

NHS Workforce

At the time of writing, there is a UK shortage of more than 100,000 NHS staff (1 in 11 posts), affecting all key staff groups. Vacancies in adult social care are rising with a current shortage of 110,000 staff, with 1 in 10 social worker and 1 in 11 care worker roles unfilled. A recent study has shown aside from gastroenterology, all clinical professions would need additional government investment between £142 and £260 million per year to meet the 45% growth ambition of the NHS cancer workforce until 2029.

International recruitment has been key in filling such vacancies and Brexit is likely to negatively affect the ability of the NHS to successfully fill these in the short term. Healthcare professionals can be incentivised to work in the UK using different tactics, e.g. joint academic appointments to promote research and innovation, cross-provider working, enrolment in aspiring leader courses, relocation packages, and schemes that promote workforce equality and diversity.

Regulation of Medicines

Prior to Brexit, the UK had been a member of the European Medicines Agency (EMA) which provides market authorisation for new medicines and gave the UK 'Tier 1' market

---

27. Well, we think it should. It could turn us into over self-reflective hypochondriacs.

status. This meant global pharmaceutical and medical device companies prioritised the UK as a market for launching products. Now the UK's Medicines and Healthcare products Regulatory Agency (MHRA) must take on the role of the EMA, and not just national authorisations, otherwise the UK may lose its 'Tier 1' status.

Brexit risks the UK supply chain of existing medicines, radioactive isotopes, devices for patients, and specialist treatments such as gene therapies. About three quarters of all medicines, and just over 50% of the NHS devices, come to the UK via the EU. The future of medical supplies in the UK depends on the government's plan to facilitate delivery of regular medicine supplies from the EU. When it comes to medical devices, the UK will need to recognise those approved by the EU market which are 'CE-marked'. CE means 'Conformitè Europëenne', a mark declaring a product's manufacturer claims compliance with the directives which apply to the product. This will be replaced by the 'UKCA' mark post-Brexit.

Alternatively, the NHS may be 'better off' after Brexit, due to the removal of the strict competitive tendering process when it comes to NHS procurement; facilitating the movement towards ICSs, which can buy in bulk for 1 million plus people. The rapid establishment of the NHS's C19 vaccination programme may not have been possible if we were still in the EU. Nonetheless, it is vital the UK retains its capability to trade with the EU, the USA, and other countries, after Brexit.

Research and Clinical Trials
Research and clinical trials may be compromised following Brexit, given the possible restrictions on free movement of researchers across Europe and the ability to secure funding. Between 2007 and 2013, the UK received 8.8 billion euros from the EU for research and development. And NHS organisations benefitted from EU funding schemes such as Horizon 2020 and the European Structural Investment Fund (ESIF). If the vision of the government for the NHS is to be realised, there needs to be more investment, and freedom of movement for the research and academic workforce. There will also be a need for revised clinical trials regulation, to ensure sponsors are still attracted to the UK.

NHS Long Term Plan 2019
NHS Long Term Plan Explained
The LTP advocates optimisation of out-of-hospital care as follows:
1. The NHS will be redesigned to reduce pressure on emergency hospital services
2. People will get more control over their own health, with alternative care options to hospital and primary care
3. Primary care and hospital outpatient care will become digitally enabled to increase attendances, reduce unnecessary appointments, optimise remote monitoring of chronic illnesses and prevent hospital admissions
4. NHS organisations will focus on evaluating and improving population health (rather than just hitting targets), which will be linked to commissioning of services through ICSs.

The clinical priorities of the NHS will be based on peoples' demand for services, as follows:
- Children and young people - 'Saving Babies Lives Care Bundle' will roll out in maternity units
- Cancer - Diagnose 75% of cancers at stage 1 or 2 by 2028; roll out rapid diagnostic centres, faster diagnostic standards (28 days), personalised care for all
- Cardiovascular disease - Lifestyle changes and primary prevention
- Stroke - Lifestyle changes, primary and secondary prevention
- Diabetes - Remote glucose monitoring, and digitally enabled care
- Respiratory Disease - Reduction in risk factors, especially lifestyle changes
- Mental Health - Reduce inequalities in access to care
- Outpatients - Digital access to consultations and remote monitoring with reduction in hospital and GP attendances. This has been accelerated by C19.

The structure of the NHS will move away from local health organisation control (CCGs), with ICSs providing leadership for planning and commissioning care for their communities.

Prevention and Health Promotion

The NHS health risk reduction priorities for the next 10 years include: smoking, obesity and poor diet, high blood pressure, alcohol and drug misuse, air pollution, and lack of exercise. Integrative Medicine takes a 'whole person' or 'holistic' view of patients and does not focus on just treating disease. For example, a prescribed exercise and nutritional regime, along with mind-body techniques, could form part of future healthcare.

Additionally it has been shown that 'wellbeing approaches' (e.g. relaxation and music therapy) can reduce premature death in both a healthy and diseased population. Measuring population health through PROMs and PREMs will be key to understanding what does and does not work.

Digitally Enabled Care

The NHS is on the way to a digital transformation[28], from the establishment of EPRs, to the use of decision support tools and Artificial Intelligence to increase diagnostic accuracy and efficiency. Remote patient monitoring in long-term illness will be digitally enabled, along with continuous life data monitoring through wearable devices and point-of-care home kits, e.g. in diabetes, oncology, nephrology, and rheumatology. Data security and ensuring patient privacy and confidentiality is part of the challenge for digital transformation.

Future of NHS Hospitals

The combination of social prescribing, a digitally enabled NHS, and ICSs will enable patients to be treated in the right place, at the right time. For example, the traditional

---

28. Hence this book has a whole chapter on it. We could have had traditional chapters (e.g. GP, surgery or medicine).

'come to the hospital' model is no longer 'fit for purpose'. Streamlined protocols and patient initiated follow-up arrangements mean decisions about whether to treat patients as inpatients, outpatients or remotely, will be clearer.

Staff roles are changing within the hospital environment. Advanced Clinical Practitioners (many previously nurses, paramedics, or pharmacists), Physician Associates and Advanced Nurse Practitioners are now assessing and treating patients, often independently of doctors. Additionally, nurses and physician associates are being trained to provide a vascular access service in some hospitals - traditionally a medical role.

The separation of elective and emergency care to maintain essential planned surgical procedures, whilst managing over-capacity in EDs and acute wards, is starting to happen. For example, Northumbria has an *emergency care* only hospital. 'One-stop clinics' where patients can self-present or be referred and have a full work-up of investigation prior to assessment, will speed up diagnosis and treatment. This will require some reorganisation of estates, and a multidisciplinary workforce to meet the needs of the service.

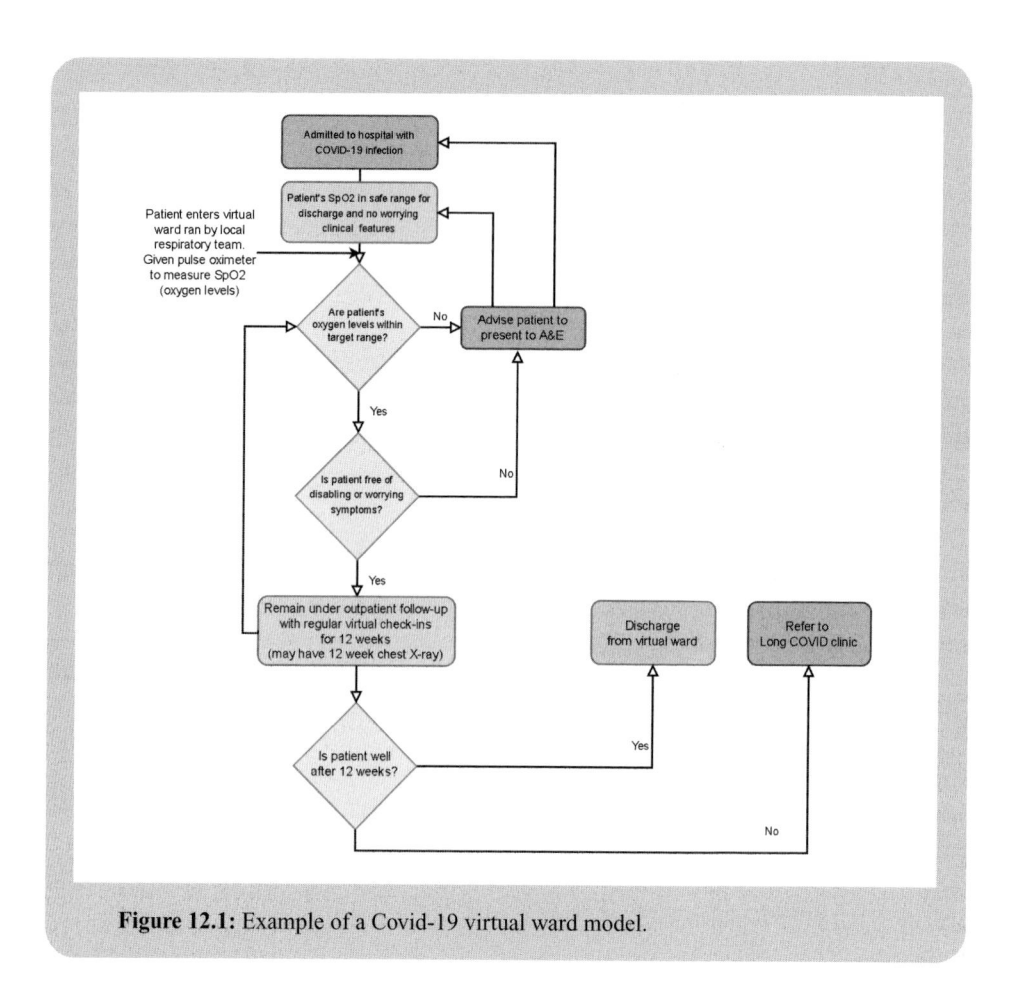

Figure 12.1: Example of a Covid-19 virtual ward model.

The C19 pandemic has accelerated the use of telemedicine within hospitals. Innovative solutions to manage bed capacity such as 'virtual C19' wards, i.e. managing quite sick patients remotely at home, using pulse oximetry, have been used to great effect. These facilitate safe discharge and readmission in the event of deterioration as shown in Figure 12.1.

Future of General Practice

General practice is, by far, the largest branch of British medicine. According to the Royal College of GPs, 90% of patient healthcare contacts are with their GPs who act as the gatekeepers of hospital care. A growing and ageing population, with complex health conditions, means personal and population-orientated primary care is central to the country's healthcare system. As a BMJ headline put it:

> "If general practice fails, the whole NHS fails."

But like the rest of the NHS, general practice will need to change in the future.

One example of change was the introduction of PCNs in 2019. They have been offered new funds to invest in new services to improve the health of the communities they serve. PCNs will hopefully increase the range of services available in communities.

Staff roles are changing in general practice as well. Physicians Associates assess and treat more straight forward patients independently of doctors; receptionists do triage and decide which patients need to talk to a GP; paramedics are doing home visits. As Primary Care Networks (PCNs) form, patients may have access to jointly employed physiotherapists and counsellors. Clinical pharmacists are starting to see patients after triage at the GP reception desk, with their clinical notes visible to the patient's GP.

The C19 pandemic has resulted in patients requiring support in the community long after recovering from the 'acute' phase of illness, e.g. physiotherapy, rehabilitation and mental health support, or 'Long COVID' care. PCNs will serve the purpose of managing the care of chronically ill patients in the community, including those with 'long COVID'.

The C19 pandemic has encouraged some PCNs to work flexibly and innovatively, using digital technology to enable patient triage, virtual consultations, and shared records. These changes are considered positive by GPs and (many!) patients alike and are likely to continue post-pandemic.

Lessons from Accountable Care Organisations

The term 'Accountable Care Organisations' (ACOs) is used in the USA to describe a model like the ICS in England, see Figure 12.2. ACOs are formed when healthcare providers join and are contracted to deliver all the care for a defined population for a certain period. Those providers include hospitals, general practices, private clinician associations or virtual clinicians. The goal is to provide the most appropriate cost-efficient care with patients proactively managed in the community, reducing hospitalisation and overall care costs.

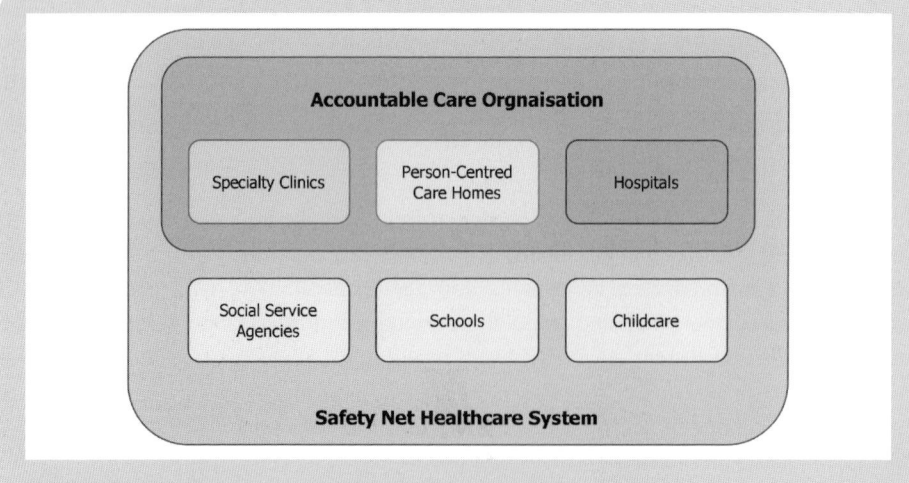

Figure 12.2: An illustrative example of an Accountable Care Organisation and overarching Safety Net Healthcare System.

ICSs will have similarities. The success of ICSs in the UK relies to a large extent on a robust 'Integrated Governance' framework. This includes data protection, as well as shared clinical pathways, policies, and procedures.

Future of Research & Development

The UK National Institute of Health Research (NIHR) and Clinical Research Networks (CRNs) were set up in 2006 to Improve the Health and Wealth of the nation. Since then - with 15 active CRNs and approximately 6,100 studies per annum – the UK has been exceedingly attractive to sponsors. This initiative has also led to training 100,000 staff in research, and funding a large workforce pool. The vision of the NIHR for research is for 1 million people to be taking part in clinical research by 2023-24.

Research can solve problems in health policy and systems and, as Jonker (2018) found:

"there is significant correlation between the level of participation in interventional research studies and high CQC ratings/lower mortality rates in hospitals".

Research is, and will continue to be, an important aspect of the NHS because it raises standards and creates choices. In addition, the systematic collection of Real-World Evidence used as a research method may supersede lengthy and expensive clinical trials.

Future of Finance of Healthcare
Increased Cost
Healthcare is becoming more expensive due to:
- An enlarging population
- An ageing population with more complex health needs

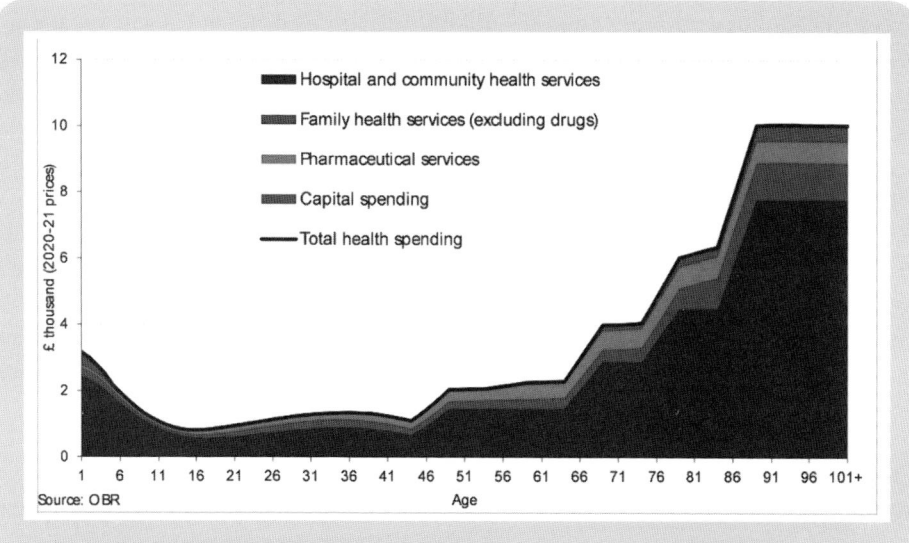

Figure 12.3: Healthcare spending per capita by age group per year (source: OBR, Health spending per person).

- Increasing expectations of the public, including what they believe should be provided by the NHS
- Increasing incidence of cancer, cardio- and cerebro-vascular disease (in frail patients, often with dementia) requiring expensive treatments and hospitalisations
- New, and more expensive, drug treatments and technologies.

Figure 12.3 demonstrates these issues.

Opposing Factors

What is interesting, and difficult to resolve, is that preventing illness and disease by reducing risk factors, e.g. smoking, can increase the long-term costs of healthcare because people live longer. For example, if we stop someone dying of a smoking-related myocardial infarction, they may live long enough to acquire another chronic condition, e.g. diabetes or cancer, which can be expensive to treat.

Some expensive drugs have been provided to the NHS at a reduced cost from the pharmaceutical industry, through managed access schemes or the Cancer Drug Fund. In addition, the voluntary sector has been supported by the government to provide services for high profile diseases such as cancer.

The advent of the internal market in the early 1980s had opposing effects on the cost of healthcare. On the one hand, the separation of purchaser and provider, led to competition both between providers and with the private sector. The idea was that competition between NHS providers would drive costs down, leading to a fairer allocation of resources. As the internal market is now being slowly (and quietly) dismantled, this idea may not (in retrospect) have been true. Or it was true, but its effect was hidden within this following issue.

On the other hand, in secondary care, as each episode of care is individually funded this creates a perverse desire to over-investigate, over-treat and build empires by 'looking for' new patients, new work, and set up new services. This may be more influential than the internal market, as demonstrated by the continued rise in NHS costs.

Economic Evaluation

Healthcare professionals should be trained in how to perform simple economic evaluations. A cost-benefit analysis, for example, will examine the cost of a resource, comparing it to value of the benefit or outcome. 'Return-on-Investment' (ROI) is another measure to demonstrate cost vs benefit; as can a 'Cost Effectiveness Analysis' (CEA). Both compare the cost of the resource to the clinical benefit of the intervention, enabling comparison between interventions.

Quality Measurement

The NICE preferred measure of clinical benefit in economic evaluation is the QALY (Quality Adjusted Life Year) because QALYs take into account both length of life and quality.

Personalised Care Packages

Personalised Care Packages (PCPs) and Personalised Health Budgets (PHBs) could also be introduced over the next few years. The benefits of PCPs include the assurance of effective and equitable care provision, as well as the rationing of expensive resources through economic evaluation. Clinical prioritisation of resources can be done by comparing the cost effectiveness of interventions.

Maintaining a High-Quality NHS Service

To ensure a high quality of care is maintained in the current volatile and uncertain world, there needs to be a robust NHS governance framework. Key performance metrics must be specific, measurable, and adaptable. Simplicity is also key, so all health workers feel they can affect them.

The NHS of the future must adopt a culture of continually evaluating and improvement, to ensure high customer satisfaction and better outcomes. A fundamental example in the UK are the CQC's five 'Key Lines of Enquiry' (KLOEs), which form the basis for all provider inspections, and are continually refined to reflect the changing needs of the NHS and social care. The five KLOEs are: Safety (protecting patients from harm); Effectiveness (providing evidence-based care); Caring (treating patients with respect); Responsiveness (to patient needs); and Good Leadership (accountable leaders). We believe they can continue to play a pivotal role in shaping the future NHS.

Public-Private Partnerships (and Lessons from Covid-19)
Workforce
Proponents of public-private partnerships argue they should not be seen as equivalent to privatisation, but as a move towards improving the quality of health services and

contributing to public education. The C19 pandemic showed this to be - at least in part - true as the NHS was shown to be part of a larger system in which collaboration with the private sector was beneficial. For example, the private sector was vital in the rapid development of new treatments, investigations (such as PCR testing), vaccines (e.g. the Astra-Zeneca vaccine), and providing sites for planned cancer and other important cold operations.

Partnership between the public and private sector has been suggested as a means of sharing knowledge and skills, as well as enabling clinical training, networking and access to new therapies and technologies. For example, such a partnership has been developed during the C19 pandemic, leading to on-going independent sector contracts with the NHS for the continuation of essential cancer surgery.

Research
Public-private partnerships are particularly important in promoting research. In 2000, the UK NHS Plan proposed financial incentivisation to reward collaboration between primary/secondary/tertiary medicine and the social and private sectors, to enhance public research capability. In 2016, KPMG found most research funds in the UK, in the year 2000, came from the private sector (£3,000m), followed by the voluntary sector (£540m) and the DHSC.

In 2006, the NIHR system was established, to partner with universities, NHS institutions, private providers, patients, and the public - for the purpose of delivering high quality research. This led to the rise of the Academic Health Science Networks, which are strongly linked to NHS hospitals, and are key to the implementation of the future NHS research strategy.

Conclusion
The future NHS requires action to create a model that is aligned with the overall healthcare strategy of the UK and is acceptable to the people it serves - whilst controlling the level of healthcare spending - in a post-Brexit, post-Covid UK.

At the time of writing, there are opportunities for sustainable change in healthcare provision. This should benefit government, health organisations - and, most importantly, patients. In such a volatile and unpredictable world, it is more important than ever to reflect on what the NHS has achieved over the years, and how the NHS and its staff have adapted to rapid change, e.g. during the C19 pandemic. We have shown ourselves to be nimble, with the ability to change according to the needs of the day. We need to use that learning to adapt, survive, and innovate during future challenges, e.g. Brexit, other pandemics, or whatever else may come.

To make the NHS the best healthcare system in the world is possible. Digital and technological innovation will support this effort and shape the care of the future - but they are not enough on their own. Integration with geographical alignment, innovation and research, must flourish and be brought to the bedside. ICSs (with EPRs to bind them) should bring the NHS closer to industry, academia and the public. A world-leading NHS will attract a high-calibre workforce to enable it to become *the* global employer and healthcare provider of choice.

The C19 pandemic helped break up some of the organisational silos that frustrate us all. It led to greater flexibility of working, nimbleness through re-deployment, and new research with a shift of focus towards lifestyle and well-being. Certainly, more people are going for daily walks than ever before! It has also accelerated innovation that would have probably taken years to adopt and implement. This provides a unique opportunity for the NHS to maintain this momentum.

Whatever the future may hold, it is more important than ever, as you enter training as a health professional, that you are driven by what the NHS is all about: a deep commitment to helping the sick, disadvantaged and vulnerable in society. To carry that out, we need innovative thinking to develop new models of care, a diverse and talented workforce, and strong personal values and clinical leadership. That leadership will include you.

Further reading

Jonker and Fisher: The correlation between National Health Service trusts' clinical trial activity and both mortality rates and care quality commission ratings: a retrospective cross-sectional study. https://doi.org/10.1016/j.puhe.2017.12.022.

King's Fund: Accountable Care explained.

https://www.kingsfund.org.uk/publications/accountable-care-explained

KPMG: On the value of the NIHR network.

https://www.nihr.ac.uk/documents/partners-and-industry/NIHR_Impact_and_Value_report_ACCESSIBLE_VERSION.pdf

NHS: Breaking down barriers to better health and care.

https://www.england.nhs.uk/wp-content/uploads/2019/04/breaking-down-barriers-to-better-health-and-care-march19.pdf

Chapter 13

Glossary and Acronym-Buster

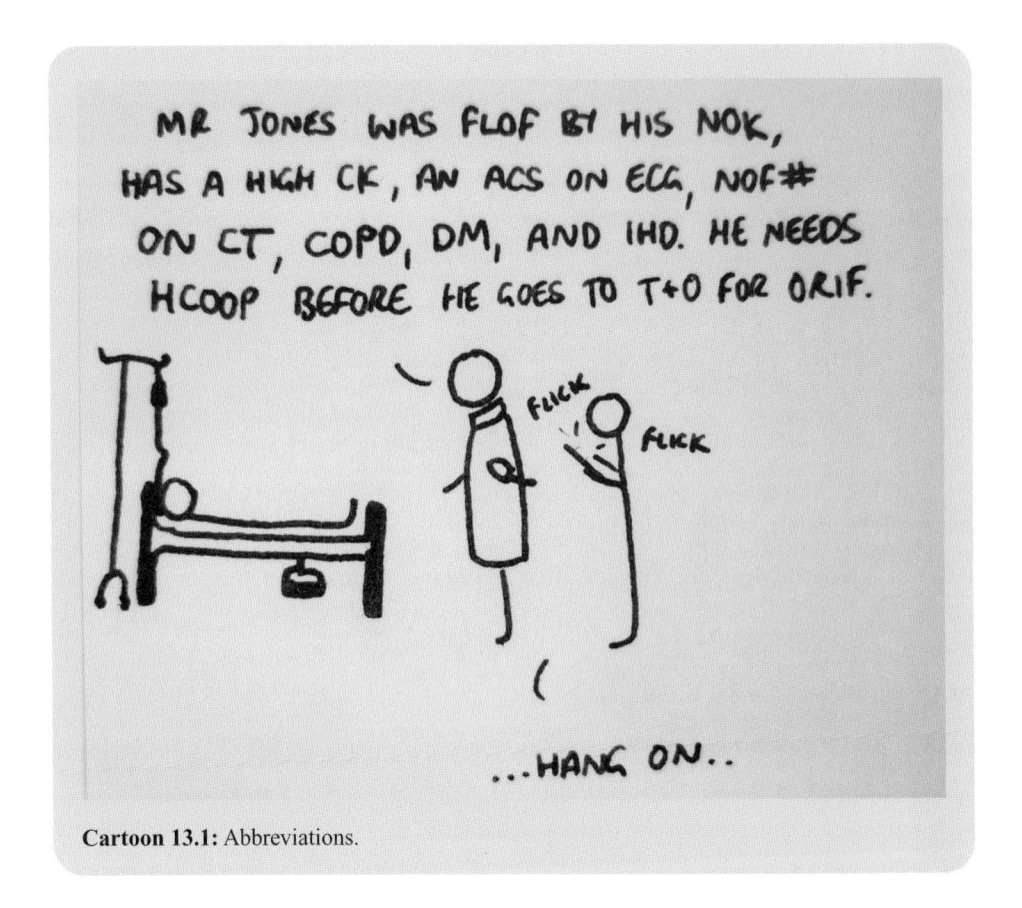

Cartoon 13.1: Abbreviations.

2 Week and **31/62 Day Cancer Targets:** In England when a GP suspects cancer, at least:
- 93% should see a hospital consultant within 'Two week wait' (TWW)
- 96% should wait no more than 31 days from receiving diagnosis and 'decision to first treatment'
- 85% should wait no more than 62 days from original urgent GP referral, to have 'first definitive treatment'

4 Hour Emergency Care Target: Known as '4 Hours', expects 95% of emergency patients to be seen, treated if necessary, and either discharged or admitted, within four hours from arrival at emergency department (ED)

12 Hour Trolley Wait: Patient should not wait to be admitted on a trolley (for e.g. in the ED or an ambulance) for over 12 hours. Clock starts at time of decision to admit

18 Week Elective Care Target (Referral to Treatment: RTT): Maximum waiting time for non-urgent, consultant-led treatment in NHS (e.g. a hip replacement) from GP referral. Also known as '18 weeks'

111: NHS non-emergency number

1948: NHS was established on the 5 of July 1948

999: Official emergency telephone number in UK. Allows caller to contact emergency services (police, ambulance, fire and others) for urgent assistance

Top Tip (999, When to Ring). This should only be used in an emergency. If the situation is serious and needs rapid (but not urgent) medical help, ring 111 (or use the NHS 111 website)

A

A&E: Accident and Emergency: Now more commonly called 'ED' (Emergency Department)

AAU: Acute Assessment Unit. Also called **Observation** or **Short Stay Ward**

AC: Audit Commission: Appoints, set the standards for and oversees auditors working in range of local public bodies in England

ACO/S: Accountable Care Organisation/System: Integrates and merges funding of primary and secondary care (and ideally social care); providing incentives to keep people healthy and out of hospital

ACP: Advanced Clinical Practitioner

Acute Care: Medical, surgical or psychiatric treatment usually in hospital

Acute Hospital: A District General, Teaching (Medical) or Psychiatric (Mental Health) Hospital which delivers acute and chronic treatments

Admission: Process of admitting a patient to hospital

Admission Rate: Number of people admitted to hospital per unit time

Admitted Pathway: Care patient receives once admitted to hospital

Advice and Guidance: Encrypted email system whereby a GP can ask a hospital consultant for advice, e.g. whether to refer or not

ADR: Adverse Drug Reaction

Advocate: Someone who supports people and acts on their behalf

AEC/AECU: Ambulatory Emergency Care/Unit: Unit for medical (non-surgical) patients who can be treated with short-term emergency care as an **Outpatient.** See **SDEC**

AfC: Agenda for Change: NHS grading and pay system for staff, except doctors, dentists, apprentices and some senior managers

AHA: Area Health Authority: 'Area': Previous 'sub-regional' NHS area of administration/finance in England. Approximately size of **STP/ICS** (i.e. covering 1 million people). There were 90

Alongside Midwifery Unit: Midwifery birthing unit on same site as obstetric service

Ambulance Targets (NHS): Ambulances should respond to Category 1 calls in 7 minutes on average, and 90% in 15 minutes

AMHP: Approved Mental Health Professional: Replaced ASW role in 2007 and applies to all health and social care professionals approved to work with people with mental health issues

AMU: Acute Medical Unit

AO: Accountable Officer: Usually Chief Executive Officer, i.e. most senior person responsible for care delivered by an organisation. See **CEO**

AOT: Assertive Outreach Team

Appraisal: Formal assessment of performance of an employee

AQP: Any Qualified Provider: Commissioning approach allowing any provider who can provide specific service and meets the required minimum standards, to apply. Patients can choose which provider on AQP List they wish to see. See **AWP**

ASW: Approved Social Worker: Started in 1983 – can work with people with mental health issues

Attendance (hospital): Attendance of individual at hospital or ED

AWP: Any Willing Provider: Any organisation suitable to tender for NHS contract. See **AQP**

B

BAME: BME: Black, Asian and Minority Ethnic: Black and Minority Ethnic

Banding: NHS has nine pay bands for non-medical staff, see **AfC**

Bank Nurse: Nurse who works occasional shifts

BAU: Business As Usual

BC: Business Continuity: System of management (BCM) giving an organisation a framework for identifying and managing risks that could disrupt normal service

BCF: Better Care Fund: Funding from DHSC for local NHS organisations and councils to work together to plan and deliver integrated care

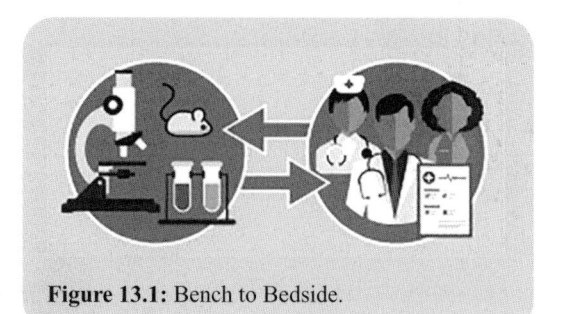

Figure 13.1: Bench to Bedside.

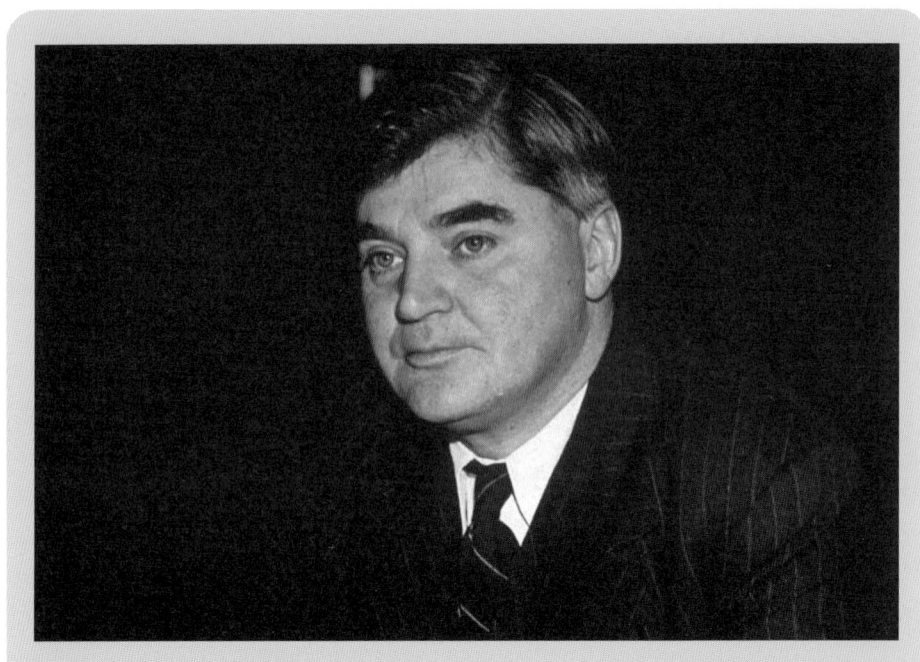

Figure 13.2: Nye Bevan MP.

'Bench to the Bedside': Process by which results of research done in laboratory are directly used to develop new ways to treat patients

Benchmarking: Comparing performance to best standards, practices or averages

Bevan, Aneurin (1897-1960): 'Nye Bevan', a British Labour politician, considered the 'Father of the NHS'

Block Contract: Process by which Purchasers agree with Providers a fixed budget for a certain period

BNF: British National Formulary: Book detailing all medicines used in the UK

Board: Group of people who supervise activities of an organisation (e.g. Hospital or CCG), usually led by a **Chairperson** who supervises a **CEO**

Broker: Someone who helps patients (and families) choose a Nursing or Residential Home

C

C4C: Case for Change: 'Management speak' describing a reason for policy change

CAE: Clinical Adverse Event: Patient Safety Incident that could have caused (a 'near-miss'), or did result in, harm to people or groups of people. See **Datix**

CAG: Clinical Advisory Group

Caldicott Guardian: Senior person responsible for protecting confidentiality of service-user information and enabling appropriate information sharing

Call to Action: Sets out request to patients, public, staff and partners to join a national conversation about future demand on NHS services

CAMHS: Child and Adolescent Mental Health Services

Capital: Spending on land, premises and equipment

Capitated payments: Package of funding allocated to service 'provider' based on number of people registered with them, e.g. GP funding

Care Leavers: Any adult who spent time in care as child

Carer: Family member or paid helper who regularly look after another person

CC: Community Care: Health or social care services provided to patients in and around their home

CCG: Clinical Commissioning Group: Local level of NHS administration/finance in England

CD: CL: Clinical Director: Clinical Lead: Head of hospital department (or small group of). Usually a doctor

C diff: Clostridium Difficile

CDU: Clinical Decision Unit

CEO: CFO: Chief Executive Officer: Chief Financial Officer

CFH: Connecting for Health: Maintains and develops NHS national IT infrastructure

Chaplain: A faith leader who can arrange access to leaders of most faiths

Chairperson: Senior person on a **Board** of organisation

CHC: Continuing Healthcare: NHS Continuing Healthcare: Care outside of hospital, e.g. in nursing home, funded by NHS for people whose care needs are predominantly health related

Children's Act: Allocates duties to local authorities, hospitals, courts, police and parents, and other agencies, to ensure children are safeguarded

Choice: Process whereby patients can **Choose and Book** their preferred hospital and/or clinician

Choose and Book: Computerised system by which GP and patient can exert **Choice** over which hospital/clinician the patient is referred to

CI: Commissioning Intentions: Proposed plans to purchase services

CIO: Chief Information Officer: Senior person responsible for information technology and computer systems

CIP: Cost Improvement Plan: Identifying, delivering and monitoring cost improvement programmes

Clinical Audit: Systematic, critical analysis of quality of care (e.g. diagnosis or treatment), use of resources, or outcome for patients

Clinical Governance: System through which staff/organisation(s) are accountable for continuously improving quality of service

Clinical Guideline: Provides guidance (local, national or professional) about pathway (e.g. investigation) or treatment

CMHT: Community Mental Health Team

CMO: Chief Medical Officer: Senior doctor in organisation

CMT: Clinical Management Team

CST: Core Surgical Trainee: Stage of a hospital doctor's training between **FY1/2** and **ST: Specialty Trainee.** Previously called 'SHO' (senior house officer)

CNO: Chief Nursing Officer

COG: Chief Officers Group

Commissioning: Process of planning, buying and monitoring health services

Commissioning Support Units (CSUs): Provide support and services for CCGs such as finance, HR, data management, or contracting

Community Matron: CM

Community Nurse: Provides nursing care in community settings

Competition: Following passing of the HSC Care Act 2012, NHS Providers must compete with private companies for contracts to provide NHS funded services

Consent: Permission required from patient before any test or operation

Consultant: A senior hospital-based doctor who has completed all their specialist training and placed on their speciality's Specialist Register

'Contracting Out': Where the NHS purchases services from private sector, charities or other bodies

COO: Chief Operating Officer: Usually second most senior manager in management team, reports to CEO. Responsible for the day-to-day running of organisation

Coronavirus: Group of RNA viruses causing variety of diseases in humans and other animals. They include **COVID-19**

Coroners Court: Inquires into causes and circumstances of some deaths

COVID-19: C19: Respiratory disease caused by SARS-Cov-2. 'CO' stands for corona, 'VI' for virus, and 'D' for disease. Caused 2019-2022 pandemic

CPA: Care Programme Approach

CPD: Continuing Professional Development: How health professionals continue to learn and develop throughout career

CPN: Community Psychiatric Nurse

CPR: Child Protection Register

CPR: Cardiopulmonary Resuscitation

CRHT: Crisis Resolution and Home Treatment team: Supports people with mental health problems in community

CQC: Care Quality Commission: Inspector and regulator of health and social care in England

CQUIN: Commissioning for Quality and Innovation: Payment mechanism enabling commissioners (e.g. a CCG) to reward (financially) excellence

CSSU: Children's Short Stay Unit

CVS: Community and Voluntary Sector

D

DASS: Director of Adult Social Services

DAAT: Drug & Alcohol Action Team

Data Protection Act 2018: Controls how personal information used by organisations

Datix: Computerised system used to collect and store **CAE**s

Day Case: Having operation or procedure, and going home same day. See **DSU** and **SODA**

DCS: Director of Children's Services

Department (hospital)**:** Hospitals divided into departments of different branches of medicine, and grouped into **Divisions** (or **Directorates**)

Departmental Manager: Manager who runs department

DGH: District General Hospital: Local smaller hospital

'DH': Department of Health: Previous name for **DHSC**. Originally Ministry of Health

DHA: District Health Authority: 'District': Former local level of administration/finance of the NHS in England. Later became PCT/PCG then CCG. There were 192

DHSC: Department of Health and Social Care: Government department leading health and social care

Discharge: Process by which patient leaves hospital

Discharge Lounge/Hub: Where patient waits to be picked up to go home

Discharge Summary: Summary of patient's hospital stay sent to GP. See **e-DS**

D2A: Discharge-to-Assess: Process used to enable early discharge from hospital, by AHPs assessing patient's longer-term needs in home

District Nurse: Community-based nurse

Division (or Directorate): Grouping of **Departments** in hospital

DNA: Did Not Attend: As in an appointment

DNACPR: Do Not Attempt Cardio-Pulmonary Resuscitation. See **ReSPECT Form**

DNAR: Do Not Attempt Resuscitation. See **ReSPECT Form**

DNR: Do Not Resuscitate. See **ReSPECT Form**

DoLS: Deprivation of Liberty Safeguards: Allows short-term withdrawal of liberty from people that are a danger to themselves

DoS: Directory of Services: List of services hospital or general practice provides

DPO: Data Protection Officer

DPH: Director of Public Health

DQ: Data Quality

Dr: Abbreviation of doctor

Dr Foster Intelligence (known as '**Dr Foster**'): Provider of computerised monitoring of NHS performance. Sends alerts to hospitals if it 'sees' increase in mortality or morbidity

DRE: Delivering Race Equality

Drug and Therapeutics Committee: Produces local formulary (list) of approved drugs

DSU: Day Surgery Unit. Also called **SODA.** See **Day Case**

DTC: Diagnosis and Treatment Centre

DToC: Delayed Transfer of Care: Delayed from when patient is ready to leave hospital

DUP: Duration of Untreated Psychosis

Duty of Candour: Healthcare professionals must be honest when something goes wrong

E

E&D: Equality and Diversity

Early Adopter: Person or organisation who starts (or pioneers) using a new health system

EAU: Emergency Assessment Unit

EBH: EBM: EBP: Evidence-Based Healthcare: Medicine: Practice

ED: Emergency Department. See **A&E**

EDD: Expected Date of Discharge

EDM: Electronic Document Management

e-DS: Electronic Discharge Summary: See **Discharge Summary**

Education Outcomes Framework: Used by **HEE** to measure education, training and workforce development

EHR: Electronic Health Record

EI: Early Intervention: Coordinated services supporting families during early childhood

EIP: Early Intervention to Psychosis

Elective Care: Pre-arranged, non-emergency care e.g. scheduled operations. See **Planned Care**

EOC: Elective Orthopaedic Centre

EoLC: End of Life Care

EPR: Electronic Patient Record

e-portfolio: Electronic portfolio of evidence

e-prescribing: Computer-based system for prescriptions

e-referral: Electronic method of referring patient

EqIA: Equality Impact Assessment

Escalation of Care: Process recognising and acting on clinical deterioration

ESR: Electronic Staff Record

Executive Team: Very senior managers in organisation

Expert Patient: Patient with a chronic disease whose knowledge empowers them to play a part in their management and treatment

F

Family Planning: Use of contraception

Family Therapy: Type of psychological therapy

FBC: Full Business Case

FCE: Finished Consultant Episode

FHS: Family Health Services

'Firm': Previous term for group of doctors that work with particular consultant or ward

FOI: Freedom of Information

Follow-up: Second or subsequent appointment

Freedom to Speak Up: Process that supports staff if they have concerns about care

FRG: Finance Review Group

Friends and Family Test: Asks patients if it would recommend their service to a loved one

FT: Foundation Trust: Type of not-for-profit hospital independent from DHSC

FY1/2: Foundation Year 1 and 2: First- and second-year post-qualification doctors. Also known as 'F1s' and 'F2s'. FY1/F1 previously called 'House Officer'

G

Gap Analysis: Comparison of actual with desired healthcare performance

GDPR: General Data Protection Regulation: Regulation meaning care data will be handled securely. Part of the Data Protection Act 2018

General Practice: A place where GPs work

GMS: General Medical Services: A type of GP contract

Governance: 'Rules' governing internal conduct of organisation by defining staff roles and responsibilities

GP: General Practitioner: A general (family) doctor

GP Federation (or Association): Group of General Practices working together

GPOOH: GP Out-of-Hours: GP services offered outside normal working hours

GP Safe Haven: Surgeries where GPs can safely see potentially violent patients

Group Manager: Hospital Departmental Manager

H

HCA: Healthcare Assistant: Support nurses. Also called **Nursing Auxiliary** and **Support Worker**

HCAI: Healthcare-associated infection

HDA: Health Development Agency: Forerunner of **NICE**

Health: Defined by WHO as 'a state of complete physical, mental and social well-being and not merely absence of disease or infirmity'

Health and Social Care Committee: UK Government Committee that examines the running of the **DHSC**

Health and Wellbeing Board (HWB): Set up by **HSC Act 2012** bringing together representatives from CCG, local Healthwatch and local authority, to understand local community's needs and identify commissioning priorities

Health Boards: Scotland, Wales and Northern Ireland run through regional health boards

Health Commission: NHS inspectorate, 2004 to 2009, then incorporated into the **CQC**. Evolved from Commission for Health Improvement (CHI)

Health Inequalities: Differences in health state or status between individuals or groups

Health Professional: Person qualified in healthcare services

Health Record: Patient's care record

Health Systems Support (HSS) Framework: Helps NHS organisations access support services from innovative suppliers

Healthwatch England: Statutory body whose sole purpose is to understand needs, experiences and concerns of people who use health and social care services, and speak on their behalf

HEE: Health Education England: Responsible for healthcare education in England

HEMS: Helicopter Emergency Medical Service

HES: Health Episode Statistics

HFEA: Human Fertilisation and Embryology Authority: Regulates and inspects clinics in the UK providing in vitro fertilisation, artificial insemination and storage of human eggs, sperm or embryos. Also regulates human embryo research

HMSR: Hospital Standardised Mortality Ratio: Measures whether number of deaths in a hospital is higher or lower than expected. See **SHMI**

'House': Previous term for new team of junior doctors every 6 months (now 4 months)

HPA: Health Protection Agency: Former agency who protected public in England from infectious diseases and environmental hazards

HR: Human Resources

HRA: Health Research Authority: Responsible for protecting interests of patients in health research and streamlining research regulation

HSC Act 2012: Health and Social Care Act 2012: Provided for extensive reorganisation of structure of NHS in England

HSE: Health Survey for England: Yearly survey monitoring nation's health and care

I

IAPT: Improving Access to Psychological Therapies: Team of mental health workers providing therapy to people with mild mental health problems

ICAS: Independent Complaints Advocacy Service: Independent NHS complaints advocacy service organised by local authority

ICD-11: Eleventh revision of International Classification of Diseases

ICO: Information Commissioner's Office

ICS: **Integrated Care System:** Integrates primary, secondary, community and other health and care services in to one entity, under one single contract, developed out of **Sustainability and Transformation Partnership (STP)**. See **ACS/O**

IFR: Individual Funding Request

IG: Information Governance: Ensures appropriate use of personal information

IMCA: Independent Mental Capacity Advocate

IMT: Internal Medicine Trainee: Stage of a hospital doctor's training between FY1/2 and ST: Specialty Trainee. Previously called 'SHO' (senior house officer)

IMHA: Independent Mental Health Advocate

Independent Sector: Voluntary, charitable and private care providers

Information Department: Collects information for health professionals

Inpatient: Someone admitted and staying in a hospital

Integrated Care: Bringing together delivery, management and organisation of services related to clinical care, rehabilitation and health promotion

IPS: Individual Placement and Support

ISVA: Independent Sexual Violence Advisors / Advocates

ITT: Invitation to Tender

J

JAG: Joint Advisory Group

JCVI: Joint Committee on Vaccination and Immunisation

JHWS: Joint Health and Well-being Strategy

JSNA: Joint Strategic Needs Assessment: Written yearly by local **Health and Wellbeing Board**s, regarding current and future health and care needs of local population

K

King's Fund: A 'think tank' exploring how healthcare can be improved

KPI: Key Performance Indicator: Target agreed between purchaser (commissioner) and provider concerning performance of a service

L

LAS/LAT: Locum Appointment for Service/Training: Temporary contract for registrar-level doctor

LDP: Local Delivery Plan: Plan to show how CCGs make improvements

Lean Thinking: Business methodology about how to organise activities to deliver more benefit and value, whilst eliminating waste

LETB: Local Education and Training Board: Regional group (or 'deanery') of **HEE**

LLoS: Long Length of Stay: Excessive stay in hospital. Not defined but often taken to be over 14 days (average LoS is under 7 days)

Local Authority (LA: council): Local government. Responsible for social care

Local Health Number: Identification number provided by a hospital, in addition to an NHS Number. See **NHS Number**

Locum: Having temporary contract

LoS: Length of Stay: Time patient stays in hospital

LPA: Lasting Power of Attorney

LTA: Long-term Agreement

LTC: Long-term Condition

M

MADE Event: Multi Agency Discharge Event: Used to 'get a hospital flowing' by encouraging patient discharges. Usually a week long

MAU: Medical Admission Unit

MCA: Mental Capacity Act 2005: Legal framework for making decisions on behalf of adults who lack capacity. See **IMCA**

MDT: Multi-Disciplinary Team

'Medical' (as in 'Have a Medical'): Assessment of general health/screening

Medical Director: Most senior doctor in organisation. See **CMO**

Medicines and Healthcare products Regulatory Agency (MHRA): Regulates medicines (including vaccines), medical devices and blood components for transfusion in UK

Mental Health: Person's psychological and emotional well-being

Mental Health Act 2007: Covers care and treatment of mentally disordered persons, in England and Wales

Mental Health Nurse: Nurse who specialises in mental health

Mental Health Targets (NHS): 75% of people referred to **IAPT** programmes should begin treatment within 6 weeks of referral, and 95% within 18 weeks

MHIT: Mental Health In-Reach Team

MIU: Minor Injury Unit

MLU: Midwife-Led Birthing Unit: Maternity unit staffed and usually run by midwives

MMT: Medicines Management Team: Team providing evidence-based approach to prescribing balancing safety, tolerability, effectiveness, cost and simplicity of treatments

MOC: **Model of Care:** Overarching design for particular type of healthcare service shaped by evidence-based practice and defined standards

Modern Matron: Experienced nurse who runs **Department** in a hospital. They should be visible, accessible and focused on improving experience of patients

Monitor: Former NHS body that monitored finances of Foundation Trusts. Became part of **NHS Improvement** in 2016

MRSA: Methicillin-resistant Staphylococcus Aureus: A 'super-bug' and used as marker of hospital hygiene

MUPS: Medically unexplained physical symptoms

N

NAO: National Audit Office: Scrutinises public spending on behalf of Parliament

National Tariff: Nationally agreed price for procedures or activities

NCEPOD: National Confidential Enquiry into Patient Outcome and Death

Figure 13.3: NHS sign.

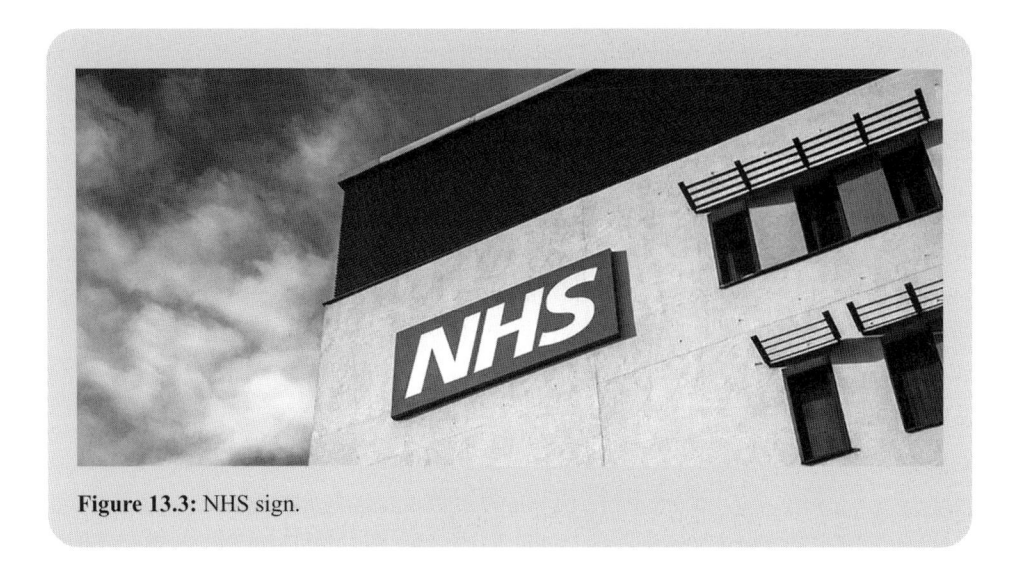

NCVO: National Council for Voluntary Organisations: Umbrella body for voluntary and community sector in England

NED: Non-Executive Director: Director without day-to-day responsibility for organisation who sits on **Board**

Never Event: Very serious **PSI** (Patient Safety Incident) that is preventable

NFR: Not for Resuscitation

NGO: National Guardians Office: For Freedom to Speak Up Guardian

NHS: National Health Service

NHSX: Unit with oversight of digital strategy and policy in **NHSE**

NHS Business Services Authority: NHSBSA

NHS Blood and Transplant: NHSBT: Co-ordinates blood products and organs for transplantation

NHS Commissioning Board Authority: Transitional body for **NHSE** October 2011 to April 2013

NHS Complaints Advocacy: Free, confidential service available to anyone who wants support to make complaint

NHS Confederation: Membership body for organisations commissioning and providing NHS services

THE NHS CONSTITUTION
the NHS belongs to us all

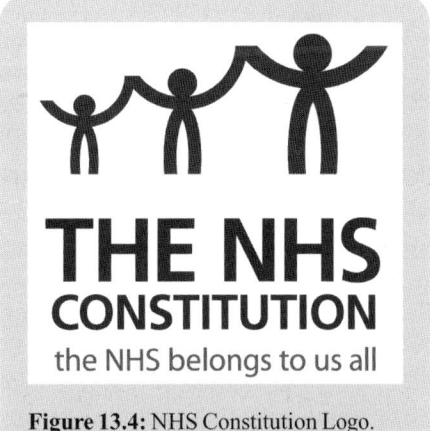

Figure 13.4: NHS Constitution Logo.

NHS Constitution (for England): The principles, values, rights and responsibilities underpinning the NHS

NHS Counter Fraud Authority: Formed in 2017 to identify, investigate and prevent economic crime

NHS Digital: National information and technology partner for health and care systems. Supports organisations to get best out of technology, data and information

NHS Employers: Help employers develop a sustainable workforce and improve staff experience. Part of **NHS Confederation**

NHS England: NHSE: Runs the NHS in England

NHS England Lead Provider Framework: Enables CCGs, NHSE and others to access support; ranging from back-office operations to services driving long-term transformation

NHS England Region: 'Region': NHS England divides the nation into 7 administrative regions: East of England, London, Midlands, North East and Yorkshire, North West, South East and South West. See **Sub-Region**

NHS Evidence: Part of **NICE** and a resource of research information

NHS Executive: Defunct (1995-2002) national NHS management executive

NHS Improvement: NHSI: Responsible for overseeing NHS hospitals in England, as well as independent providers providing NHS-funded care, now merged with **NHSE**

NHS Improving Quality: NHSIQ: Part of NHSE, set up to support improved health outcomes

NHS in Northern Ireland, Scotland and Wales: Devolved Healthcare

NHS Information Centre: NHSIC

NHS Key Skills Framework: NHSKSF: Defines and describes knowledge and skills NHS staff need

NHS Leadership Academy: Training organisation ensuring NHS leaders are developed

NHS Litigation Authority: Manages claims against NHS in England

NHS Low Income Scheme: Provides financial support to people who may be entitled to full or partial help with prescriptions, dental and other treatment, if they have a low income

NHS Number: A number that you are given when you are born. It is expressed as 3 groups of numbers, like this: 123 456 7891. See **Local Health Number**

NHS Prescription Services: Responsible for NHS drug prescriptions and appliances, and payments to dispensers in England. Part of **NHSBSA**

NHS Research Authority: NHSRA: Research regulator which protects and promotes interests of patients and public in health and social care research. See **RES**

NHS Resolution: Provides expertise to **NHS** on resolving concerns fairly and sharing learning to improve patient care

NHS Supply Chain: Manages procurement of healthcare products, services and food for NHS organisations across England and Wales

NICE: National Institute for Health and Care Excellence: Independent organisation providing guidance on health promotion and prevention, and treatment, of ill health

NICU: Neonatal Intensive Care Unit

NIHR: National Institute for Health Research

Non-Elective Care: Care for people needing urgent treatment for acute illnesses

Non-PbR: Non-Payable by result: Activity based on reference costs

Notifiable Disease: One which the law requires to be reported to authorities

NPSA: National Patient Safety Agency: Former monitor of **PSI**s

NQB: National Quality Board: Provides coordinated leadership for quality on behalf of national health bodies, e.g. **DHSC**

Nuffield Trust: 'Think tank' exploring how healthcare can be improved

Nursing Associate: New role withing nursing team. Work with **HCA**s and **Registered Nurse**s. Similar to **SEN**

Nursing Auxiliary: NA: Also called **HCA** and **Support Worker**

Nursing Home: Accommodation with nursing care

NSF: National Service Framework: Defunct long-term strategies for areas of care

O

Observation Ward: Also called **AAU** or **Short Stay Ward**

'One Stop' Clinic: Efficient outpatient model designed to allow consultation, diagnosis and treatment to happen, at one outpatient appointment

ONS: Office for National Statistics

OOHC: Out-of-Hospital Care

OPD: Outpatient Department or simply 'Outpatients'

Operational Team: Usually synonymous with **SMT**

OOH: 'Out-of-hours': Outside normal working hours, i.e. 9am-5pm, Monday-Friday

Outpatient: Patient who comes to a hospital service not for admission

P

PA: Programmed Activity: 4h unit of work used to determine consultant's pay

Package of Care: PoC: A combination of services put together to meet a person's health and social needs

Pandemic: Disease, usually infectious, prevalent over a whole country or world

PACS: Picture Archiving and Communications System: Digital x-rays

PALS: Patient Advice and Liaison Service: Offers confidential advice, support and information on health-related matters

PAS: Patient Administration System: Records patient's demographics and contact with hospital, both **Outpatient** and **Inpatient**

Pathway: Process of diagnosis, treatment and care

PAU: Paediatric Assessment Unit:

PbR: Payment by Results: System that sets fixed prices for clinical procedures and activity

PCN: Primary Care Network: Groupings of GP practices typically with patient population of 30,000-50,000

PCP: Personal Care Plan

PCSE: Primary Care Support England: Part of NHSE. Provides support services to GP Practices, Pharmacies, Dentists and Optometrists across England

PCT/PCG: Primary Care Trust/Group: Defunct local level of NHS administration/finance in England. See **CCG** and **DHA**

PFI: Private Finance Initiative: Programme to enable private sector to provide facilities (e.g. build a hospital) which will be run by NHS

PHSO: Parliamentary and Health Service Ombudsman: Government body that makes final decisions on complaints not resolved by NHS in England

Physician Associate: PA: University trained practitioner who provides supervised mid-level medical care, such as the diagnosis and treatment of common conditions

PIP: Patient Information Point

PLACE: Patient-Led Assessments of Care Environment: Self-assessments by a combination of NHS and private/independent healthcare providers and patients

Planned Care: see **Elective Care**

'Postcode Lottery': Situation in which someone's access to health services or medical treatment is determined by where they live

PPA: Prescription Prescribing Authority: Responsible for administering prescription charging

PPE: PPI: Patient and Public Engagement: Involvement

PPE: Personal Protective Equipment: Gloves, aprons, masks, etc.

PPG: Patient Participation Group

PPC: Prescription Prepayment Certificate: Yearly certificate whereby patients can pay fixed amount rather than for every prescription

Pre-op: Pre-operative Assessment: Hospital clinic where suitability for operation or procedure is assessed

Primary Care: Healthcare delivered outside hospitals

Procurement: Process of sourcing and supply of goods and services. See **NHS Supply Chain**

PROM: Patient Reported Outcome Measure: Assesses quality of care from patient's viewpoint

Provider: Healthcare organisations providing healthcare services - bought by a **Purchaser**

PSI: Patient Safety Incident

PSNC: Pharmacy Services Negotiating Committee: Promotes interests of NHS community pharmacies in England

Public Health: PH: Specialism concerned with improving health of population

Public Health England: PHE

Purchaser: Organisations that buy health and social care from **Providers**

'Purchaser-Provider Split': Creation of an 'internal market' within the NHS

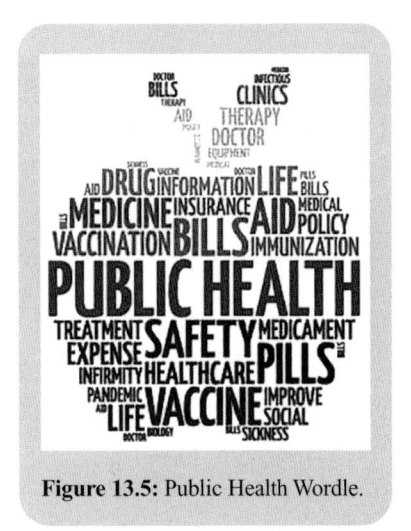

Figure 13.5: Public Health Wordle.

Q

QA: Quality Assurance

QALY: Quality-Adjusted Life Year: Used in economic evaluation to assess value of medical interventions. One QALY equates to one year in perfect health

QIPP: Quality, Innovation, Prevention and Productivity: Programme to achieve efficiency savings

Quality: Standard of something in healthcare as measured against other similar things

Quality Improvement: About making healthcare safer, effective, patient-centred and timely

Quality Premium: Financially reward for CCGs for improvements in quality

QOF: Quality and Outcomes Framework: System for performance management and payment of GPs

R

R&D: Research and Development

RCA: Root Cause Analysis: Systematic process to analyse causes of incidents and learn from them

Re-ablement: Services to maximise people's long-term independence, choices, quality of life and minimising requirement for ongoing support

Readmission: When a patient is readmitted to hospital with same condition, usually within 28 days

Reconfiguration: Rearrangement of services or facilities to achieve a benefit

Regional Hospital Board: RHB: Defunct (original) regional NHS geographical area of hospital administration/finance in England. There were 14 in 1948

Registered Nurse: Default title for all nursing registrants in UK

Registrar: A doctor in the middle of postgraduate specialty training

Reorganisation: Politically driven healthcare changes which occur periodically

RES: Research Ethics Service: Part of **NHS Research Authority**

Residential Home: Home with supervision for people who need more than just housing, e.g. elderly people, or adults with learning difficulties. See **Nursing Home**

ReSPECT Form: Recommended Summary Plan for Emergency Care and Treatment Form: A plan for recording recommendations to guide clinical decision-making in an emergency. Includes guidance on **DNAR** and **Escalation of Care**

Revalidation: Process by which regulatory bodies confirm continuation of professional's licence to practise in UK

RHA: Regional Health Authority: 'Region': Previous regional NHS area of administration/ finance in England. There were 14

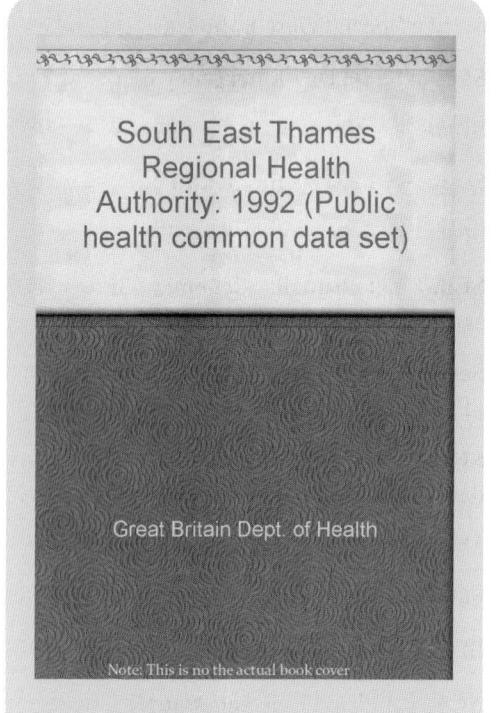

Figure 13.6: Example of Document produced by SE Thames RHA.

Risk Management: Identifies circumstances which put patients, carers and staff at risk of harm and then acts to prevent or control those risks

RSU: Regional Secure Unit: Medium-secure units for people thought to pose special risks, particularly of violence

RTT: Referral to Treatment: Time taken for patient to be referred by a GP to the start of an appropriate (usually hospital-based) treatment (often an operation). See **18 Week Elective Care Target**

S

Safe Havens (NHS Digital): Ensure confidential patient data can be transmitted and stored securely

Safeguarding: Means protecting peoples' health, well-being and human rights, and enabling them to live free from harm, abuse and neglect

SARS-Cov-2: Virus that causes **COVID-19 (C19)**

SAU: Surgical Admission Unit: Surgical equivalent of an **MAU**

SCBU: Special Care Baby Unit: see **NICU**

SDEC: Same Day Emergency Care: Alternative name for **AEC(U)**

Secondary Care: Healthcare provided in hospital

Secretary of State for Health and Social Care: Cabinet politician who leads **DHSC**

SEN: Defunct name for State Enrolled Nurse. See **Nursing Associate**

SES: Single Equality Scheme: Strategy and action plan detailing a Trust's commitment and approach to equality and human rights

Seven Day Service (7DS): Provision of healthcare to an equal standard over seven days of the week

SHMI: Summary Hospital-level Mortality Indicator: Measures whether number of deaths in hospital, or within 30 days after leaving hospital, is as expected. See **HMSR**

Short Stay Ward: Also known as **Observation Ward** or **AAU**

SIGN: Scottish Intercollegiate Guidelines Network: Scottish equivalent of NICE

SITREP: Situation Report: Description of a situation, event, or incident

SLA: Service Level Agreement: Document setting out an agreement between two or more parties, describing expectations and requirements of each party

SMI: Severe Mental Illness

SMT: Senior Management Team: Some will be members of **Executive Team**

Social Admission: Person admitted to hospital as they cannot cope at home

Social Care: All forms of personal and practical assistance for people

Social Care Package: Combination of services put together to meet a person's **Social Care** needs

Social Distance: Perceived or desired degree of appropriate remoteness between people

SODA: Surgery On Day (of) Admission: See **Day Case** and **DSU**

SPA: Single Point of Access: Describes process where services share single set of contact information, e.g. telephone number, email or web address, etc

SPA: Supporting Professional Activity: Activities carried out by a consultant that underpin direct clinical care, e.g. training, **CPD**, **Clinical Audit** and **Clinical Governance**

Special Notes: Information recorded about patients with complex needs, where needs of these patients could not be met without additional information

Specialist Commissioning: When NHS commissions specialise services for rare and complex conditions, e.g. rare cancers, dialysis or cardiac surgery

Specialist Register (of **GMC**): List of doctors eligible for appointment as consultant in NHS

SRN: State Registered Nurse: Defunct name for **Registered Nurse**

SSRB: Senior Salaries Review Body: Provides independent advice to government on pay of managers (and others) in NHS

ST: Specialty Trainee: Registrar doctor in middle of specialist training

Stakeholders: People who have a 'stake' (interest) in how NHS is run, e.g. patients, staff and commissioners

STP: Sustainability and Transformation Plan/Partnership: Geographical division of England, created by **NHSE** ready to integrate their services and funding more fully. May become an **Accountable Care Organisations/System** (**ACO/S**) or later an **ICS**

Stranded/Super-stranded Patient: Patient whose **LoS** is 7 (stranded) or 21 days or more (super stranded)

Sub-Region: Administrative geographical area (and/or financial level) between a regional (currently **NHS Region**) and local (currently, **CCG**) level of control. **ICS**s will be this level

Substantive: Having a permanent contract

SUI: Serious Untoward Incident

Suicide/Parasuicide: Talking about, or attempting to, take ones' own life

Summary Care Record: SCR: Contains important information from record held by **GP**. Includes details of medicines, allergies, demographic details and NHS Number

Support Worker: Also called **HCA** and **Nursing Auxiliary**

SUS: Secondary Uses Service: Collection of healthcare data required by hospitals and used for planning healthcare, and supporting payments

T

Talking therapy / treatment: Treatments which involve individual or group sessions with trained mental health professional (e.g. counsellor or psychotherapist)

TDA: Trust Development Authority: Defunct organisation responsible for overseeing performance management and governance of Non-Foundation NHS Trusts. Became part of **NHS Improvement** in 2016

Teaching Hospital: Hospitals where medical students and doctors (and other health professionals) train; usually bigger than **DGH**

Telemedicine: Remote diagnosis and treatment of patients by means of telecommunications technology

Tertiary Care: Complex treatments for less common illness, usually in specialist centre

Transfer: Internal = moving a patient from one ward to another. External = moving a patient to another healthcare provider

Triage: Sorting patients in order of urgency to determine order of treatment, e.g. in **ED**

Trust: All NHS hospitals in England are managed by one

Trusted Assessor: Assessor of inpatients on behalf of residential or nursing homes

U

UCC: Urgent Care Centre: Often GP – led, they offer patients access without an appointment. See **UTC** and **Walk-in Centre**

UKHSA: United Kingdom Health Security Agency: Successor to Public Health England

Unconscious Bias (Medical): Attitudes or stereotypes unconsciously affecting medical understanding, actions, and decisions

Urgent Care: Another name for **Non-Elective** (or Emergency) Care

UNA: Unable to Attend: Patient unable to attend an appointment vs **DNA** (Did Not Attend)

UTC: Urgent Treatment Centre: **Walk-in Centre** or **UCC**

V

Values: Important precepts which guide behaviour

Vanguard Sites: Organisations chosen to lead development of new care models

VCS: Voluntary and Community Sector

VCSE: Voluntary, Community and Social Enterprises

Virtual clinic: Clinics held over phone, video or internet. Used widely in C19 pandemic

VTS: **Vocational Training Scheme:** A training scheme for GPs

W

Waiting List: List of people waiting to see a doctor, or an investigation, procedure or operation (usually non-urgent). Because of NHS targets (mainly **RTT**), this should not be excessive (should be under 18 weeks)

Walk-in Centre: Another name for **UCC** or **UTC**

Ward: Place in a hospital where **Inpatients** are looked after

Ward Clerk: Staff member who deals with day-to-day administrative running of the ward

Ward Manager: Senior nurse in charge of hospital ward

Ward Round: When a group of health professionals visit an inpatient, usually led by a senior doctor (**Consultant** or **Registrar**), with junior doctors and nurses in attendance

Weekend Effect: Excess morbidity and mortality (11%) related to less effective healthcare delivered at the weekend

Whistleblowing: Policy and mechanism representing the **Freedom to Speak Up** when staff see something wrong happening

WLI: Waiting List Initiative: Extra work undertaken to reduce waiting lists

Wrong Site Surgery: Surgery performed on wrong patient or wrong part of body e.g. wrong knee

WTE: Whole time equivalent: WTE of 1 is equivalent to an individual working full time; and 0.5 WTE is part time, at half the hours

X, Y, Z

YTD: Year to date

'Yellow Form' (BNF): Form used to report **ADR**

Zero Length of Stay: Patient is admitted to hospital and leaves within 24 hours

Chapter 14

History of NHS Summary

	Legislation	Government	National	Regional	Area	Local	GP	Other
1848			General Board of Health (GBH)					
1858			GBH abolished					
1911	National Insurance Act 1911						GPs developed lists ('panels') of patients	
1919		Ministry of Health (MoH)						
1948	Creation NHS - National Health Service Act 1946		Central Health Services Council (CHSC)	14 Regional Boards	147 Local Health Authorities (LHAs)		138 Executive Councils	388 Hospital Mx Committees (HMCs), 36 Boards of Governors (Teaching Hospitals)
1968		MoH becomes part of Department of Health and Social Security						

217

	Legislation	Government	National	Regional	Area	Local	GP	Other
1974	National Health Service Reorganisation Act 1973			14 Regional Health Authorities (RHA)	90 Area Health Authorities (AHA)	192 District Health Authorities (DHA)	90 Family Practitioner Committees (FPC)	FPCs coterminous with local authorities
1982					AHA abolished			
1983			Health Services Supervisory Board (HSSB)					
1985			NHS Management Board					
1988		Department of Health (DHSS splits) to become Department of Health (DoH) and the Department of Social Security (DSS)						
1990	NHS and Community Care Act 1990						Fund-holding GPs (FH GPs)	FPCs became Family Health Services Authorities (FHSAs)
1995	Health Authorities Act 1995		NHS Executive (NHSEx)	8 NHSEx Regional Offices		95 Health Authorities		

History of NHS Summary

1996								National Specialised Commissioning Group (NSCG)
1999							481 Primary Care Groups PCGs, abolishing FH GPs	FHSAs incorporated into PCGs; NICE formed
2001	Health and Social Care Bill 2001			28 Strategic Health Authorities (SHA)		17 Primary Care Trusts (PCTs)		
2002		NHSEx abolished, becoming 4 NHSEx Directorates						
2003		4 NHSEx Directorates abolished						
2005			4 committees of CHSC abolished			303 PCTs		
2006				10 SHAs, from 28		152 PCTs		
2007								National Specialised Commissioning Team (NSCT); CQC formed
2011				4 SHA 'Clusters'				

219

	Legislation	Government	National	Regional	Area	Local	GP	Other
2012								HEE formed
2013	Health and Social Care 2012		NHS England (NHSE)	4 NHSE Regions		PCTs replaced by 211 Clinical Commissioning Groups (CCGs)		NHSE regions include specialised commissioning teams Public Health England, Healthwatch England and Health & Wellbeing Boards formed
2014					44 Sustainability and Transformation Partnerships (STPs)			CCGs merging as part of STP formation
2016								NHS Improvement formed
2018		DoH becomes Department of Health and Social Care (DHSC)						
2019				7 NHSE Regions (from 4)				

History of NHS Summary

2020					42 Integrated Care Systems (ICSs) forming out of STPs		Public Health England becomes National Institute for Health Protection (NIHP); further merging of CCGs
2021							NIHP becomes UK Health Security Agency (UKHSA)

Index

Page numbers ending in g indicate a glossary entry.

Academic Health Science Network (AHSN), 191
Accident and emergency (A&E), 9, 16–18, 20, 22, 28, 29, 155, 170, 173, 194g
Accountable care system/organisation (ACO/ACS), 187–8, 194g
Advanced clinical practitioner (ACP), 51, 54, 184, 194g
Advanced health practitioner, 53–4
Agenda for Change (AfC), 49–50, 195g
Age UK, 105
Allied health practitioner (AHP), 28, 40, 62
  See also Dietitian/dietetics, occupational therapist, osteopath, physiotherapist, podiatrist, radiographer, speech and language therapist (SALT)
Ambulance, 7, 43
  services, 154–5, 161
  technician, 67
  See also Call handler, emergency care assistant, paramedic, patient transport service
Approved mental health professional (AMHP), 107–8, 195g
Armed forces/services, 72, 75, 81
Assertive outreach team (AOT), 103, 195g

Banding, 49, 195g
Barnett Formula, 42
Bevan, Aneurin, 5–7, 33, 48, 163, 196g
Block contract, 39, 196g
British Dietetic Association (BDA), 35, 63, 85

British Medical Association (BDA), 25, 35, 85, 110
British Social Attitude Survey, 46–7
Call handler, 67
Cancer, 17, 22, 28, 38, 46, 65, 88, 90, 125–7, 180, 185
  bowel, 21
  breast, 18
  cervical, 114, 128
  lung, 8, 115, 123
  screening, 13, 21, 30
  targets, 18, 22, 170, 193
Cancer Drug Fund (CDF), 79, 189
Cardiac surgery, 9, 28, 38, 75, 88–9
Cardiology, 37, 39, 57, 87, 90, 151
Care programme approach (CPA), 72, 104, 199g
Care Quality Commission (CQC), 18, 22, 31, 72, 76, 188, 199g
Certificate of Completion of Specialist Training (CCST), 16, 85
Certificate of Eligibility for Specialist Registration (CESR), 60
Chartered Society of Physiotherapy, 63
Chemotherapy, 38, 60, 89, 94
Chief Executive Officer (CEO), 68–9, 83, 197g
Chief Financial Officer (CFO), 68–9, 197g
Chief Medical Officer (CMO), 68, 82, 198g
Chief Nursing Officer (CNO), 68–9, 82
Chief Operating Officer (COO), 68–9, 198g
Children, 53, 74, 90

Index

Children Act 1989, 108
Children's nursing, 40, 53
Children and adolescent mental health services (CAMHs), 101, 197g
Choice, 16, 21, 22, 116, 120–1, 169
Choose and Book, 148, 197g
Clinical commissioning group (CCG) 23, 30, 73, 119, 123, 197g
Clinical manager, 67–8
Clinical senate 74
Clinical priority advisory group (CPAG), 91–2
Clinical reference group (CRG), 91–2
Clinical research network (CRN), 130, 138, 188
Cognitive behavioural therapy (CBT), 59, 100
Commissioning support unit (CSU), 73, 198g
Community mental health team (CMHT), 101, 103, 198g
Court of Protection, 109
COVID-19 / C19, 17, 24, 25–6, 112, 113, 125–6, 166, 198g
    and Out of Hours care, 32–3
    lessons from, 190–2
    long covid, 187
    post covid, 155–7
Crisis resolution and home treatment (CRHT) Team, 101, 102, 199g

Defence medical services (DMS), 81
Dental care training (DCT), 61–2
Dental nurse, 62
Dental hygienist, 62
Dental therapist, 62
Dentistry, 23, 28, 34–5, 60–62, 80, 170, 175
Department of Health and Social Care (DHSC), 9, 42–4, 72–3, 81, 82, 166, 169, 191, 199g
    IT strategy, 156
Deprivation of Liberty Safeguard (DoLS), 108–9
Dietitian/dietetics, 28, 62–3
Dialysis, 38, 75, 89, 95, 144, 180
Digital enabled therapy (DET), 100
Distributive justice, 121–2
DNACPR, 154, 200g

Doctor, 40–42, 54–5, 61, 67, 76, 83, 88, 154, 163–4, 175
    See also Junior doctors, medical school, physician, registrar, surgeon
Dr Foster Intelligence, 14, 18, 19, 79, 200g

Electronic patient record (EPR), 147, 155–6, 168, 181, 185, 201g
Emergency Care Assistant, 67
Emergency department (ED), 26, 39, 99, 193, 201g
    See also A&E
Executive director, 68

First contact practitioner, 28
Florence Nightingale, 2, 63
Forensic mental health team, 99, 101–2
Foundation training, 55, 56, 57

General Dental Council (GDC), 62, 77
General manager, 12, 67
General Medical Council (GMC), 3, 16, 19, 41, 56, 59, 72, 75
    Specialist Register, 58, 76, 87, 214g
General Medical Services (GMS) Contract, 30, 202g
General Pharmaceutical Council (GPC) 33, 66
General practice, 6, 29–31, 56, 80, 147, 160, 164, 187, 202g
General practitioner (GP) 2, 15, 27–30, 56, 87, 202g
GP Association/Federation, 31, 202g
Genome Project, 23
Group manager, 202g

Healthcare assistant (HCA), 51–2, 202g
Health and Care Professions Council (HCPC,) 62, 63, 64, 66, 70, 77
Health and Social Care Act (HSC), 2012 23, 73, 96, 204g

223

Health and Wellbeing Board (HWB), 74, 125, 203g
Health Education England (HEE), 77–8, 92, 154, 169, 203g
Health visitor, 7, 52–3, 81, 152
Healthwatch England (HWE), 10, 20, 75, 85, 203g
High-cost drug, 92
Highly specialised service (HSS), 91–2
HMSR (Hospital Standardised Mortality Ratio), 203g
  See also SHMI
Holding powers, 108
Hospital
  board, 6, 10, 39, 68, 93, 212g
  district general (DGH), 2, 8–9, 37, 199g
  municipal, 2, 5, 6
  hyper-specialist, 38
  structure, 39, 67
  teaching, 6–7, 10, 28, 38, 75, 81, 89, 93–4, 215g

Immunisation, 29, 111, 113–4, 125–6
Improving access to psychological therapy (IAPT), 18, 22, 24, 59, 99, 100, 204g
Independent Sexual Violence Advisor/Advocate (IVSA), 27, 204g
Individual Funding Request (IFR), 79, 204g
Influenza A, 17, 112
Innovation, 73, 74, 77, 83, 136, 181–2, 191–2
Institute of Biomedical Sciences accredited degree programme, 70
Integrated Care System (ICS), 31, 39, 74, 97, 103, 180–81, 204g
Integrated Research Application System (IRAS), 139, 141
Internal Medicine Training (IMT), 57

King's Fund, 192

Lasting Power of Attorney (LPA), 109, 205g
Learning disability, 53, 74, 88, 89, 90, 102, 104
Local authority, 2, 10, 42, 108, 127, 165, 205g
Local council, 2, 114, 125, 169

Manager, see clinical manager, general manager, group manager, practice manager, senior manager, ward manager
Manual for Prescribed Specialised Services, 89
Medical director, 68, 82, 206g
Medical laboratory scientific officer (MLSO), 70
Medical Register, 76
Medical school, 55–6
Medicines and Healthcare products Agency (MHRA) 20, 79, 139, 184, 206g
Mental health, 17, 18, 24, 28, 37 101–6
  Mental Capacity Act 2005, 21, 108, 206g
  Mental Health Acts 1959/1983/2007, 8, 12, 99, 101, 102, 107, 127, 06g
  mental health nurse, 53, 206g
Mental illness, severe (SMI), 38, 100, 102–3, 106, 213g
Midwife/midwifery, 52, 152, 206
Military, 40, 81, 83
Ministry of Defence (MOD), 81
Mind, 104, 105
Minor Injury Unit (MIU), 32, 121, 206g

National Cancer Registry, 125, 126
National Institute Health and Social Care Excellence (NICE), 15, 17, 41, 43m 78–9, 100, 106–7, 144, 209g
  appraisal process, 91
National Institute of Health Research (NIHR), 129–30, 137, 143, 188, 191, 209g
National insurance, 42
National Insurance Act 1911, 4, 7, 127, 217
National medical director, 24, 83
National Programmes of Care (NPoC) 90–91
National Service Framework (NSF) 15, 17, 99, 209g
National specialised commissioning group 95–6
National Tariff Payment System (NTPS), 92
Neurosurgery 28, 38, 75, 89
NHS App 25, 148, 150–51, 156
NHS Blood and Transplant, 21, 72, 207g

Index

NHS Constitution, 18, 22, 179, 181, 208g
NHS Digital, 72, 79–80, 146, 149, 150–52, 161, 168, 208g
NHS England (NHSE), 23–24, 25, 39, 42–3, 69, 72–3, 74–5, 106, 125, 152–3, 208g
   chief professional officer, 82–3
NHS England Health and Justice (NHSE HJ), 82
NHS Five Year Forward View 2014 (5YFV), 24, 74, 180, 183
NHS Health Research Authority (HRA), 129–30, 139, 141, 143, 203g
NHS Identity, 148, 149–50, 156
NHS Improvement (NHSI), 25, 43–4, 75, 80, 152, 208g
NHS Long Term Plan 2019, 25, 103, 109, 180, 184–5
NHS Mental Health Implementation Plan 2019, 102
NHS Net/Mail, 150
NHS Standard Contract, 88
NHSX, 25, 80, 148, 152, 207g
Non-executive director (NED), 39, 69, 207g
Northern Ireland, 1, 6, 7, 9, 10, 25, 34, 42, 44, 82, 84, 92, 125, 163
Nuffield Trust, 85, 93, 209g
Nurse
   Advanced Practitioner, 51, 186
   district, 28, 29, 209g
   Macmillan, 30
   Marie Curie, 30
   mental health, 53
   paediatric, 53
   practice, 28, 49
   Registered, 40, 51, 73, 211g
   School, 40
Nursing associate (NA), 51, 76, 209g
Nursing and Midwifery Council (NMC), 19, 51, 76

Occupational therapist (OT), 40, 63–4
Operating department practitioner (ODP), 65
Optician, 28, 35, 72

Optometry, 35, 75, 80
Osteopathy, 37, 62

Package of Care, 209g
PACS (Picture Archiving and Communication System), 147–8, 151–2, 156, 210g
Paramedic, 66–7
Parity of Esteem, 106
Pathology, 37, 39, 87
Patient and Public Involvement (PPI), 137, 143, 210g
Patient transport service, 67
Payment by Results (PbR), 39, 210g
Perinatal mortality, 46
Pharmacist/pharmacy, 28, 33, 54, 65–6, 72
   clinical, 187
   community, 167
Pharmacy technician, 66
Physician, 57, 180
Physician associate, 20, 53, 186–7, 210g
Physiotherapist, 28, 63, 77, 167, 186
Podiatrist, 28, 35–6, 65
Poor Law, 2
Population, Intervention, Comparison and Outcome (PICO), 134–5
Practice manager, 30, 70
Pregnancy 33, 35, 36, 52, 160
Prescribed specialised services, 89, 90
Prescription, 8, 32, 33–4, 35, 42, 62
   electronic, 146, 148, 149, 201g
   Prescription Prescribing Authority (PPA), 210g
   prescription pre-payment certificate, 34, 211g
Preventative medicine, 24, 29–30, 33, 120
Primary care, 17, 19, 27–8, 29–37, 72, 75, 80, 95, 99, 109, 147, 148, 164, 172, 184
   mental health, 100
   network (PCN), 30–31, 72, 80, 180–181, 187, 210g
   post-covid, 155
Prison, 40, 43, 53, 59, 72, 82, 101, 119
Private Finance Initiative (PFI), 18, 40, 210g
Procedural justice, 122
Professional body, 42, 72, 78

225

Provider, 13, 15, 39, 180, 189, 196, 211g
Psychiatric Intensive Care Unit (PICU), 101–103
Psychiatrist / psychiatry, 29, 38, 53, 59–60, 100–101, 107
Psychotherapy / psychotherapist, 59
Psychologist, clinical 59–60
Public and patient voice (PPV), 91
Public health, 2, 3–4, 8–17, 19–22, 23–25, 62. 72. 78, 111–28, 169, 211g
   Director of Public Health (DPH), 200g
   faculty of, 127
   Northern Ireland, 84
   Public Health England (PHE), 24, 26, 41, 72, 211g
   Scotland, 83
   Wales, 84
Purchaser, 13, 15, 39, 180, 189, 196, 211g

QALY, 190, 211g
Quality assurance, 76, 211g
Quality Surveillance information system, 91
Quaternary care, 38

Radiographer, 64
   therapeutic, 65, 172
Radiologist, radiology, 58–9, 64, 181
Rape crisis centre, 36–7
Rare Diseases Advisory Group (RDAG), 92
Recovery academies, 105
Registrar, 16, 30, 58, 59, 62, 212g
Research 16, 38, 39, 57–8, 85, 125, 129–45, 169, 184, 191
   and development (R&D), 181, 188, 212g
   clinical, 129–32
   costs, 137–8
   ethics, 138–9, 212
   funding, 135–6
   impact, 144
   questions, 134–5, 137
   types, 132–3
Royal College(s), 42, 72
   Academy of, 78
   of General Practitioners, 8, 10
   of Nursing, 84
   of Occupational Therapists (RCOT), 64
   of Physicians, 57, 123
   of Psychiatrists, 107
   of Speech and Language Therapists (RCSLT), 64
Royal Society of Medicine (RSM), 85

Scotland, 1, 6, 8, 34, 42, 44, 82, 83–4, 92, 125m 163
Screening, 126
   abdominal aortic aneurysm, 22, 40
   cancer, 13, 21, 30, 128
Secondary care, 27, 28, 37–8, 40, 80, 81, 99, 147, 183, 213g
   and IT Services, 156–9
   mental health, 100–101, 103
Senior manager, 67–8, 182, 201
Severe Acute Respiratory Syndrome (SARS)
SHMI (Summary Hospital-level Mortality Indicator), 213g
Smoking, 89, 117, 181, 189
   and cancer, 8, 123–4, 127
   cessation of, 29, 33, 40, 65, 66, 81, 118, 183
   prevention of, 109, 185
Social care, 30, 39, 42, 45, 73, 78, 81, 101, 103, 165–9, 177, 183, 190, 214g
Specialised commissioning, 43, 88–91, 95
Specialist/specialty training (ST), 16, 58, 62, 214g
Speech and language therapist (SALT), 64
Spine I/II, 147–9, 151
Strategic clinical network, 74
Summary care record (SCR), 149, 215g
Surgeon, 58, 156, 160, 180
Sustainability transformation partnership (STP), 74, 80, 214g
Syd (See yourself differently), 157

Taxation, 42, 85, 167
Telemedicine, 160, 187, 215g
Tertiary care, 27, 37–8, 80–81, 99, 101, 215g
Transplantation 28, 38, 75, 89, 92, 180

Index

Trial Management Unit (TMU), 141–3
Tuberculosis (TB), 119

UK Health Security Agency (UKHSA), 26, 112, 125–6, 215g
Unions, 85
Urgent care/treatment centre (UCC/UTC), 31, 121, 215g

Vaccination, 2, 7–8,
Vascular Surgery, 58, 160

Velindre NHS Trust, 84
Virtual assistants in healthcare (CERi), 157, 159
See also Syd
Voluntary, community and social enterprise (VCSE), 104, 216g

Wales, 6, 9, 34, 42, 82, 84, 108, 125, 163
Walk-in centre, 18–19
Ward manager, 216g